RADICAL
SISTERS

Also by Judith L. Pearson and available
from Mayo Clinic Press

Crusade to Heal America:
The Remarkable Life of Mary Lasker

RADICAL
SISTERS

**SHIRLEY TEMPLE BLACK,
ROSE KUSHNER, EVELYN LAUDER,
AND THE DAWN OF THE
BREAST CANCER MOVEMENT**

JUDITH L. PEARSON

MAYO CLINIC PRESS

The publisher wishes to thank Sandhya Pruthi, M.D., for her support and review of this book.

The medical information in this book is true and complete to the best of our knowledge. This book is intended only as an informative guide for those wishing to learn more about health issues. It is not intended to replace, countermand or conflict with advice given to you by your own physician. The ultimate decision concerning your care should be made between you and your doctor. Information in this book is offered with no guarantees. The author and publisher disclaim all liability in connection with the use of this book. The views expressed are the author's personal views, and do not necessarily reflect the policy or position of Mayo Clinic. Mayo Clinic does not endorse the brands mentioned in this work. Any references to specific products, processes, or services by trade name, trademark, manufacturer, or otherwise do not constitute or imply endorsement, recommendation, or favoring by Mayo Clinic.

Proceeds from the sale of every book benefit important medical research and education at Mayo Clinic.

To stay informed about Mayo Clinic Press, please subscribe to our free e-newsletter at MCPress.MayoClinic.org or follow us on social media. For bulk sales contact Mayo Clinic at SpecialSalesMayoBooks@mayo.edu.

Jacket design by Rebecca Lown.

MAYO CLINIC PRESS
200 First St. SW
Rochester, MN 55905
MCPress.MayoClinic.org

ISBN: 979-8-88770-237-7 hardcover
ISBN: 979-8-88770-238-4 ebook

Library of Congress Control Number: 2024056265

Library of Congress Cataloging-in-Publication data is available from the Library of Congress.

Printed in China
First printing: 2025

For the warriors and she-roes who courageously dedicated their lives to the battle against the beast.

"The doctor can make the incision, but I'll make the decision."

—Shirley Temple Black

"I have a streak of stubbornness and a loud voice."

—Rose Kushner

"I believe that one must leave the world a better place than you found it."

—Evelyn Lauder

Contents

Foreword

During my journey to make breast cancer a public health priority, I knew well the work of Shirley Temple Black, Rose Kushner, and Evelyn Lauder. We worked at a time when the word *breast* could scarcely be uttered in public, let alone printed in mass media advertising. Our paths were shaped by shared goals, but also marked by occasional differences. We competed, debated, and sometimes squabbled, but beneath it all, there was a deep and abiding respect. Though we came from different places, with different stories, our purpose united us: to lift the veil of silence surrounding breast cancer and to create a world where this disease no longer threatened the lives of women.

Shirley Temple Black, with her luminous smile and indomitable spirit, was one of the first public figures to share her personal battle with breast cancer. By speaking openly about her mastectomy in 1972, she shattered taboos and inspired countless women to seek early detection and treatment. Shirley's courage paved the way for public conversations about breast cancer, transforming fear and stigma into hope and action. Beyond her advocacy, Shirley brought the same grace she once displayed on the silver screen to her tireless diplomatic efforts and her work on behalf of cancer patients.

Rose Kushner's journey was as radical as it was inspiring. Diagnosed with breast cancer in 1974, she defied the medical norms of the time, challenging the invasive surgeries that many women endured without informed consent. Rose became a fierce advocate for patient rights, publishing groundbreaking books and articles that demanded better treatment options and a voice for women in their healthcare decisions. She taught us that knowledge is power, and she wielded it with unyielding determination to improve the lives of breast cancer patients everywhere.

Evelyn Lauder took a different approach, harnessing her passion and lending her estimable voice to a global movement. Through her leadership at the Estée Lauder Companies and her founding of the Breast Cancer Research Foundation, Evelyn raised hundreds of millions of dollars for innovative research. She taught us that beauty and compassion could coexist, that we could transform grief into action, and that with the right tools, no dream was too ambitious.

These women, like me, began their efforts when breast cancer was shrouded in silence and fear. Together, we helped to bring this disease out of the shadows, ensuring that it became a matter of public discourse and policy. Each of us knew that this work would demand more than a single lifetime. Shirley, Rose, and Evelyn dedicated their lives to this cause, working tirelessly until their final days. They left us a legacy of courage, compassion, and progress—a legacy I am honored to carry forward.

For me, this mission began in 1981, following a promise I made to my sister, Suzy, who died of breast cancer at the age of only thirty-six. I pledged to fight until we found a cure or a way to live with this disease. That promise became the foundation of Susan G. Komen, an organization dedicated to changing the way the world views and treats breast cancer. Together with our Race for the Cure series, we grew to host events in more than one hundred cities across the United States, developed the largest series of 5K runs/fitness walks in the world, and invested more than $3 billion in breast cancer research.

I was diagnosed with breast cancer in 1984. As a breast cancer survivor who endured a mastectomy, I am thankful I did not face breast cancer alone. I was lucky to be surrounded by friends and family, dedicated healthcare professionals who helped carry my burden. As any breast cancer survivor will tell you, these people are much more than family and friends—these people are co-survivors. They are pillars of strength that live the experience with us.

These experiences inform my work today with the Promise Fund, an organization that partners with Federally Qualified Health Care Centers to break down barriers to access and equity in breast cancer care. Promise Fund reaches tens of thousands of women who are uninsured, underinsured, or have limited or no access to healthcare through a public–private partnership. The organization, founded in 2018, is dedicated to applying what we know to be effective: screening and early detection save lives. Our patient navigators provide guided support for mammography and cervical screenings, as well as early detection best practices and treatment. So much of the progress being made today was made possible through the pioneering service and advocacy of brave voices inside the breast cancer movement.

As you turn the pages of this book, you will discover the remarkable stories of these women—stories of resilience, innovation, and an unyielding commitment to change. Their efforts remind us that progress is not a straight path but a series of battles, large and small, waged by individuals who dare to dream of a better world. Shirley, Rose, and Evelyn dared. They dreamed. And they delivered.

To this day, I carry Suzy's memory in my heart, just as Shirley, Rose, and Evelyn carried their own motivations and memories. Together, we built a movement that has saved lives and will save countless more. My work continues, not only for Suzy but for every woman and family touched by breast cancer. And like these incredible women, I will keep going—until my last breath—to honor my promise and ensure that the fight against breast cancer endures.

Ambassador Nancy G. Brinker,
founder of the Susan G. Komen Foundation,
founder of the Promise Fund,
global cancer advocate

RADICAL
SISTERS

Prologue

"Most surgeons in this country no longer do the radical mastectomy, the removal of the breast and the underlying pectoral muscle. Unnecessarily mutilating, it is thought."[1] It was March 18, 1985. Phil Donahue, not quite fifty years old, propped his leg up on the edge of the stage, a casual yet purposeful pose he had perfected in hosting *The Donahue Show* for nearly two decades.

"Now, the modified radical is used most often," Donahue continued. "And now steps forward another very important study suggesting the lumpectomy might be enough for many, many women. Think of the consequences of this!" He paused dramatically.

"Who had their breast removed and didn't need to? Who's reading all those pictures [mammograms], and do those guys—and they almost always are male—know what they're doing?" The audience snickered.

A graphic popped onto the screen, entitled "Breast Cancer Facts." Bullets spelled out the current state of affairs:

1. One in eleven women will develop breast cancer;
2. It is the leading cancer killer in women, and the leading cause of death for women ages 30–40;
3. The five-year survival rate is 74%. For women whose tumors are small and localized, it is 96%.

"Can you imagine if the guys had this?" Donahue asked rhetorically, suggesting that perhaps society would take notice if as many men as would fill a Boeing 747 were diagnosed with a deadly disease every day of the year.

Another graphic appeared with a list of risk factors for breast cancer. They included early onset of menstruation, late menopause, having a first pregnancy relatively late in life, increased height and weight, and family history. "Incidentally," Donahue inserted, "if you have a baby at sixteen, it reduces the incidence of breast cancer."

"Now you tell me!" shouted a woman in the audience, and laughter followed.

It was the perfect segue for Donahue to turn toward the stage, where a sober-faced Dr. Marc Lippman, head of the breast cancer section of the National Cancer Institute (NCI), and a smiling Rose Kushner, a pioneering journalist and breast cancer advocate, sat side by side. Perhaps it was that Rose* could speak about breast cancer from personal experience, perhaps it was confidence from her vast knowledge of the disease and its detection and treatment, or perhaps it was just her natural demeanor, but for the entire hour that smile never left her face. At a time when newspapers were loath to even print the word *cancer*—calling it instead "the big C"—Rose was shockingly willing to share the details of her own breast cancer treatment, live and on national television.

Cancer has terrified humans for millennia. When a 1980 National Institutes of Health (NIH) survey asked women to list their most serious health concerns, a total of 76 percent put cancer at number one (44 percent specifying breast cancer).[2] Stress, high blood pressure, and heart disease troubled only 16 percent of those surveyed. Although strides had been made against cancer since President Nixon signed the 1971 National Cancer Act, the disease still evoked specters of slow and agonizing death, bereft spouses, and parentless children. In some circles, cancer was still mistakenly thought to be contagious. It was spoken of in hushed tones, and rarely discussed in public. Consequently, it was a risk to focus an entire television show on such a scourge.

And yet Donahue had. Deftly steering the discussion like a North Atlantic sea captain, he navigated the icebergs of the era's breast cancer controversies: mammography, lumpectomy, chemotherapy, and the mother of all controversies, radical

---

* Throughout the book I have generally used first names for women and girls and last names for men on second mention. However, because this book deals with medicine, women doctors are referred to as such.

mastectomy. The standard of treatment for a century, radical mastectomies had been pioneered by Dr. William Halsted at Johns Hopkins Hospital. In the early twentieth century, Halsted amputated breasts, scraped away muscles, and hacked out bone, believing that if he got to the root of the cancer, survival chances would increase. Although the term *radical* is the Latin word for "root," it also accurately described the surgery's extreme nature; it left many women debilitated for life. And it was a procedure Rose had refused when her breast cancer was diagnosed in 1974.

"I had a modified radical," Rose explained to the audience, "the removal of the breast and axillary lymph nodes, but no muscles or bone." Smiling, she finished, "In 1974, that was as hard to get as a lumpectomy is today. And I had to go to Buffalo to get it."

She had met with and rejected eight different surgeons in her hometown, Baltimore, at the NCI, and in New York City, all of whom refused her request to leave her muscles and bones intact. She finally found Dr. Thomas Dao, 370 miles away at Buffalo's Roswell Cancer Institute. Dao was practicing exactly what Rose sought, and their medical relationship would become a lifelong friendship. While many of his colleagues found her as radical as members of the ongoing women's movement who marched in the streets protesting employment inequalities, he fully supported Rose's wishes for her surgery.

"Radical" Rose would not be silenced. She was certainly not the first woman who wanted to take charge of her own body *and* what could be done to it. Nor would she be the last. But it was a steep hill to climb. For centuries, women had been expected to be passive recipients of their medical care. They were frequently not told about the severity of any life-threatening illnesses, as it was assumed the news would be more than their "fragility" could handle.

Simply put, society dictated that it was a woman's duty to do what her doctors told her. Discussions of her health, illness, or treatments were not necessary, in the doctor's office or anywhere else. Research was not a woman's friend, either. With the exception of female-specific drugs and procedures, medical trials completely excluded women.

Donahue, still discussing the battle between doctors doing radical mastectomies and those who were taking a more conservative approach, again employed drama. "The guy with the white coat . . . says to me, 'Look . . . you're going in. Let's get it all. . . . And if we take just a little bit of your breast, and you die, your husband will sue us!'"

Rose interrupted him emphatically. "The younger women aren't buying that any longer. The older women, yes: 'Doctor, I'll put my hand in yours, do whatever you want.' The younger women—and by that I mean women under fifty—aren't putting up with that anymore."

In 1985, there was a great deal that women weren't putting up with anymore. Despite what many voices claimed, women weren't fanatics, they weren't communists, and they weren't crazy. Making up more than half of the country's population, they simply wanted to be treated in the same manner as the other half—the male half.

Change was in the wind. That was evident by Rose's smiling confidence in her convictions, and by the nods and murmurs from the all-female audience. Women were demanding to be seen *and* heard (accompanied in their demands by brave men who were secure enough to join them). Equally important was more awareness and understanding of breast cancer. Better treatment options—dare they even hope for a cure?—needed to be researched. And given the ever-climbing number of new diagnoses every year, funding for breast cancer research needed to become a priority.

Today, it is hard to imagine a time when women's health was frequently marginalized, when breast cancer wasn't discussed, when October wasn't pink. And yet that was the norm in 1985. Clearly, the time had come for a change, but first it is crucial to understand the role that women in general, and their health in particular, have been assigned over the years. A new dawn in breast cancer was on the horizon.

Rose Kushner, Shirley Temple Black, and Evelyn Lauder would play pivotal roles in what was to come. Before breast cancer entered their lives, however, each had already survived grave life events, causing them to ask the question all survivors ask: Why me?

Chapter 1

Something Else to Do in the World

The twists and turns of life often lead us down unexpected paths. On the cloudy morning of Saturday, May 1, 1915, Theodate Pope was about to follow just such a path. The dark skies did not darken her mood. A pioneering architect, she was settled aboard the sumptuous RMS *Lusitania*. The first-class accommodations she had taken for herself and her maid would be more than comfortable for the six-day crossing to Liverpool. Although war had begun in Europe a year earlier, and Germany had warned other governments and steamer passengers of possible submarine attacks on ships, the *Lusitania* was leaving America, with Americans aboard. As the United States was not yet a combatant, the passengers felt safe and secure.

Six days after the ship left its moorings in New York harbor, and eleven miles off the coast of Ireland, a German U-boat's torpedo hit it, ripping it in two. In a frenzied rush, an inexperienced crew managed to launch only six of the forty-eight lifeboats. Theodate watched and figured their chances would be better in the water. She and the maid strapped on life vests and jumped from the deck. Seconds later, the two halves of the ship sank, just eighteen minutes after the attack.[1]

The women were immediately separated in the water. Theodate was buffeted around by debris and terrified passengers, finally managing to grab a floating oar before losing consciousness. When rescuers arrived, they thought Theodate was among the dead—until another rescued passenger saw her eyelids flutter. She was one of the 764 who survived; her maid was among the 1,199 who did not.

Theodate struggled with severe survivor's guilt. Why had she been spared? What purpose could her experience possibly serve? Family friend—and famed artist—Mary Cassatt provided a powerful answer: "If you were saved, it is because you have something else to do in this world."[2]

The little girl known for dimples and tap dancing was letting Hollywood down: Shirley Temple was growing up. Even her trademark curls were evolving. Precisely fifty-six in number, those curls had been carefully curated by Shirley's mother as a symbol of innocence and childhood purity.[3] Now the twelve-year-old was experimenting with styles more in line with her age.

Shirley had been born with unusual talent. She possessed a captivating screen presence and a natural flair for singing and dancing. In the early era of films, movie production moved much more quickly than it would later in its history. Consequently, from Shirley's film debut at the age of three in 1931—and to her delight—only a few weeks passed between the completion of one film and the exhilarating beginning of another.

By 1940, however, Shirley's parents (who served as her managers) felt her future films should take a different direction. This was not a discussion 20th Century Fox studio head Darryl Zanuck wanted to have. He had a "child star" under contract, not a soon-to-be teenager. Their negotiations were made even more difficult in light of the heavy shadows still hanging over Shirley's most recent movie, *The Blue Bird*.

Set in Germany during the Napoleonic Wars, the film had been an adaptation of a play by Maurice Maeterlinck. The movie's plot follows a grumpy little girl—an unusual character for consistently sunny Shirley—who goes off in search of happiness with her little brother. Their dog and cat accompany them, having been transformed by a fairy into human form. The children magically visit both the past and the future.

The bizarre storyline was overshadowed by what happened elsewhere on the first day of shooting, September 1, 1939. That was the day another German war began as Hitler invaded Poland. Exactly one week earlier, *The Wizard of Oz* had been released. The similar plot of Dorothy and a cast of other characters also wandering a strange land caused some in Hollywood to whisper that Shirley had opted to do the film in retribution for not being cast as Dorothy, though she had been considered before Judy Garland won the starring role.[4]

A much darker shadow fell on the movie toward the end of shooting. Four-year-old Caryll Ann Ekelund played the role of Shirley's as-yet-unborn little sister. Caryll Ann introduces herself, followed by an incongruous and haunting line in her wistful little voice: "I won't be with you for long." Two weeks later, a Halloween jack-o'-lantern set fire to Caryll Ann's dress. She died from the burns, stunning the cast and crew.[5]

Still, producer Zanuck had no choice but to hope for box office success with the film's January 1940 release. Seeking advance publicity, he scheduled a Christmas Eve radio broadcast, performed before a live audience as part of the radio anthology series *Screen Guild Theater*. Zanuck had secured Studio 21 in the CBS building on East 52nd Street, which could accommodate an audience of three hundred along with a symphony orchestra. The program was built around Shirley performing a scene from *The Blue Bird*, followed by a duet of "Silent Night" with the popular and talented baritone Nelson Eddy. Despite waking up with a sore throat on show day, Shirley was determined to go on with her radio debut.[6]

Shortly before her curtain call, Shirley was standing at the window of her second-floor dressing room looking down at the parking lot. While her mother was busy styling Shirley's hair, the young actress noticed a shabbily dressed woman, carrying a large handbag, who was looking into the building windows. When the woman glanced up and saw Shirley, her eyes widened in recognition and then grew angry. She shook her fist at the girl, shouting something unintelligible.

"What's she doing?" Shirley asked her mother. Without acknowledging the stranger, Mrs. Temple lowered the blinds and told Shirley to keep practicing her lines. But before the show began, Mrs. Temple's motherly instincts led her to notify theater officials. They, in turn, reported the incident to the police, who then contacted the FBI.[7]

Backstage, twenty minutes later, Shirley had completely forgotten about the woman. When the house lights dimmed and Nelson Eddy introduced her, she stepped up to the microphone to resounding applause.

The audience quieted, and she spoke her prepared line: "Thank you, Mr. Eddy. What do I do now?"[8]

"Well, anything you say, Shirley," Eddy replied. "It's your program. But if I might make a suggestion as one singer to another, how about a song?"

"All right, Mr. Eddy, I'll sing 'Some Day You'll Find Your Blue Bird.'"

The orchestra played the introduction, and as she smiled out over the audience, Shirley's gaze fell on the first row, directly beneath her. There sat the strange woman, looking every bit as menacing as she had from the parking lot. Again mindful that the show must go on, Shirley began to sing.

"Someday, you'll find your bluebird. Wait your turn . . . bide your time. . . . For when you find your bluebird, life will be . . . so sublime."

Between the short phrases, a soprano chorus incanted, "Woo-ooo-ooo." It was during these pauses that Shirley noticed shadowy figures coming slowly down each of the side aisles. She also saw the woman reach into the large handbag and remove something. Shirley Temple might have been a sheltered child, but she knew the impending danger of a handgun when she saw one. There was nowhere to hide; the only thing between her and the woman was the slender microphone stand. The unaware orchestra kept playing, and with a combination of professionalism and innocence, Shirley moved into the spoken part of her performance.

"It may be right near you, or may be worlds apart. When love comes, you'll find it on the windowsill of your heart."

As the chorus volume increased, Shirley could now see that the figures moving closer down the aisles were dressed exactly like the movie versions of FBI agents. Shirley waved her arms like a deranged scarecrow to signal them to the front row, her singing voice going flat from the exertion.

"And then you'll hear your bluebird . . . sing a song . . . of happiness . . . to you."

The woman was now standing and pointing the gun directly at Shirley. Then, inexplicably, she paused. In that split second, the men saw her and stumbled roughly over the front-row patrons to tackle her.

The following day, the FBI reported a mystifying story to Mr. and Mrs. Temple. The woman claimed that at the very moment Shirley was born, her own newborn daughter had died. She had concluded that Shirley had stolen her baby's soul and that killing her was the only way to set the soul free. Her pause before pulling the trigger spared Shirley from becoming one of the 396 homicides occurring that year in New York City. But why had the woman paused? The reason, as Shirley later said, "was hers to answer and mine to bless."

⁓

When filming began for *The Blue Bird* on September 1, 1939, there were fifty-seven thousand Jews living in Austria, a fourth of the number who had lived there just a few years before.[9] Among them was the Hausner family: Eisig, Mina, and their only child, three-year-old Helga Evelyn.

Vienna had been a vibrant epicenter of medicine, the arts, and fashion. Eisig Hausner fit right in. Dapper and intelligent, he spoke German, English, Hebrew, and Russian, along with his native Polish. He was also a businessman, owning and operating the Wiener Werkstatt (Viennese Workshop), a ladies' boutique selling delicate lingerie and the stylish hats that Mina designed. But Eisig had become anxious about Hitler's rise to power in Germany and the ensuing aggression toward the Jewish population there and in neighboring Austria. His anxiety increased with the Anschluss—the Nazi occupation of Austria on March 12, 1938.

More anti-Jewish events occurred in 1939, including the passage of the Decree for the Reporting of Jewish-Owned Property in April. It was time for the Hausners to flee Austria. Eisig was torn, however, between trying to get out of Europe altogether and going back to Poland to rescue his parents, his brothers, and their families. Mina was resolute, telling him that while she couldn't stop him from going to Poland, she and Helga would not, under any circumstances, go with him. They, Mimi stated firmly, were going to America.

By this time, their store, the family apartment, and many other belongings had been seized by the Nazis, although Eisig had hidden some silver to use in exchange for money, if needed. But an odd ally in their plan to flee had already taken care of the necessary fees.

As much as Austria's Jews felt they had to leave, the Nazis wanted them out even more—and wanted the property they would leave behind. The Nazis had established the Central Agency for Jewish Emigration to accelerate the forced emigration of Jews. Its head was Nazi officer Adolph Eichmann, who would soon become one of the major figures behind the Holocaust. Because the costs of their emigration had to be paid by the Jews themselves, Vienna's Jewish organizations appealed for financial help from other European countries and the United States. While that money did get the Jews out, it also enriched the Nazis and drained the resources of Jewish communities.

When Eisig filed his family's initial emigration documents at the agency in July 1939, he reported that he had no income and no assets, but they did have passports that were valid for one year. Mina's cousin Betty had emigrated to England the year before, so Eisig listed that country as their destination. From there, they would figure out how to get to America.

The British had become wary of the possibility that large numbers of immigrants might arrive indigent, so potential occupations also had to be listed on the documents of anyone wishing to seek safety there. Although Eisig and Mina had experience as shopkeepers, requests for such positions were always denied. Domestic service jobs, however, were plentiful, so Eisig indicated that they would be taking jobs in that capacity. Emigrants also needed to be sponsored. The Hausners were paired with a Cheltenham, Gloucestershire, couple, Colonel and Mrs. King-Harman, who paid for the family's exit visas.[10]

But bureaucracy was a Nazi specialty. Eisig was required to complete form after form, each at separate appointments, days and weeks apart. On September 3, 1939, just two days after Hitler's invasion of Poland, France and England declared war on Germany. The first step of a Nazi plan—the one that would ultimately be called the "Final Solution"—began a month later. Slowly at first, Jews who couldn't or wouldn't leave Austria were moved to Poland. The Nazis theorized that if they were gathered into a single territory, the next parts of the "solution" would be easier to accomplish.

Eisig and Mina were desperate to get out, and waiting for final approval to emigrate was agonizing. Beginning under the veil of darkness the night of November 9 and continuing until the predawn hours of the tenth, a synchronized destruction of Jewish synagogues, homes, businesses, and schools took place throughout Austria and Germany in what came to be known as Kristallnacht, the Night of Broken Glass. Nearly one hundred Jews were killed and over thirty thousand were arrested and sent to concentration camps.

Finally, a week after Kristallnacht, the Hausners' papers arrived. Their itinerary would take them via boat train to the coastal city of Antwerp, Belgium, six hundred miles away (that country was just months away from itself being invaded by the Nazis). In Antwerp, they would board a ferry to cross the English Channel to Dover. It sounded simple. It turned out to be anything but.

Tens of thousands of emigrant Jews were flooding into Belgium in the closing weeks of 1939. While a small number—like the Hausners—were only moving through the then-neutral country, many stayed, feeling they would be safe from persecution. Unable to confirm the emigrants' intentions, the Belgian government felt the only option was to ship all of them back to wherever they had come from. That was precisely what was about to happen when Eisig, Mina, and Helga were taken off the train at one of the stops.[11]

From a detention center where new paperwork was being prepared to return them to Austria, Eisig desperately wired Mina's cousin Betty for help, as Betty was working for a Welsh Member of Parliament. That MP wired the Belgian authorities that the Hausners were coming to England to live near relatives. His pleas were helpful, and the Hausner family silver further helped to expedite their release; after several agonizing hours, the family was allowed to continue their journey to England.

By 1940, they were living in Cheltenham. But their peace would be short-lived. While fighting continued on much of the European continent, the United

Kingdom was certain that Hitler would eventually turn his sights to the island nation. And the British were reminded of the enemy sympathizers and spies who had taken refuge in the country during World War I. This prompted Prime Minister Winston Churchill to move proactively. The country's aliens were divided into three classes. Those in class C were initially regarded as "friendly" and not a threat to the country. As a Pole, Eisig fell into that class.

The British further reasoned that spies would most likely be found among those who spoke German. But there was no way to discern who was actually German and who was Austrian, nor who among them might be spies. So all fourteen thousand German-speaking adults in England were rounded up, Mina among them. Since her passport identified her homeland as Austria, she was slotted into class B. Class A was reserved for the five hundred women who had identified themselves as *Reichstreue,* allying with the Nazi government. Despite Eisig's appeals and Helga's tears (she remained with Eisig), on May 30, 1940, Mina was herded off to the internment site, the Isle of Man.[12]

A self-governing British possession in the Irish Sea, the island had long been a resort destination. Now it provided a convenient and secure location for a prison. Nine camps were created to house the ten thousand men who were detained, while two camps were created on the other side of the island for the four thousand women.

There were a number of flaws in this system. The most obvious was that the classifications were mostly self-reported and relied on honesty, a quality not typically found in a spy. Furthermore, it was decided that because they were *Reichstreue,* they should be separated from the others to prevent riots. Since the majority of detainees were Jewish, it is likely that many Nazi sympathizers were placed in rooms with Jewish women, the very group they sought to eliminate.

The women were housed in resort hotels. Mina was assigned to the Ballaqueeney Hotel in the town of Port St. Mary. The only bright spot was that her cousin Betty—who also had been swept up—was interned at the other women's camp in the town of Port Erin. The two towns could have been ordinary coastal villages had it not been for the barbed wire surrounding them. Nonetheless, the women were allowed to go to the beach, work as seamstresses, and open bank accounts.

Still, Mina was terrified. She had no idea how long she would be there, or what would happen to her husband and daughter in that time. Meanwhile, Eisig was beside himself with worry. He wasn't allowed to visit Mina, but he could send letters. She could respond—though she was allowed to send only two missives weekly, limited to twenty-four lines each. And then, as quickly as the internment had been organized, there was news that the "enemy aliens" in Class B would be released.

In preparation, Eisig visited the U.S. consulate in London on July 30, 1940, only to find that their passports had expired. He was therefore denied travel visas, although the consulate did take his application for identity cards and exit permits, and promised to find them the necessary American sponsor. Eisig took a flat in the city, and much to Helga's dismay, he had to temporarily place her in a residential nursery so he could go collect their belongings from Cheltenham. When he returned, he was greeted by a very angry daughter—and by the happy news that a sponsor had been found for them in Newark, New Jersey. All Eisig needed now were their travel visas and his wife.

The visas arrived on September 9, two days after "Black Saturday," the day the Nazis began the Blitz. For forty nights, the "lightning war" systematically rained death on London, with waves of Luftwaffe bombers accompanied by fighter planes.[13] By the time Mina was finally released, on September 15, parts of London were already piles of rubble. Via the BBC, Prime Minister Churchill told his compatriots that Hitler had "resolved to break our famous island by a process of indiscriminate slaughter and destruction." As would become the custom, Churchill's words served as a battle cry to rally the citizens.

Still, the night raids caused rampant fear. They were not just a physical act of destruction but also a deliberate psychological tool. When the air raid sirens sounded, Londoners roused from their beds and fled to the nearest shelter. For the Hausners, that meant leaving their flat and running to the basement of a nearby church. Dashing through the church's graveyard, little Helga was intrigued by the snapdragons growing among the gravestones. On every terrifying dash, Mina would let her quickly pick just one. Then, snuggled on her cot in the church basement, Helga would squeeze the flower's face and its "mouth" would snap open and closed. The snapdragons provided a distraction from the cataclysm going on aboveground. And, like most Londoners, the Hausners learned the difference in sound between the British and German plane engines. When the latter flew over, they held their collective breaths, listening to the whine of the bombs before the explosions' concussions shook the basement floor.[14]

In one night alone, London authorities estimated 450 fatalities, with another 1,500 residents injured. Eisig, Mina, and Helga had already escaped so much. It would have been such a cruel twist of fate if they had died amid this chaos. But they did not.

Eisig was finally able to arrange for them to travel to Glasgow, Scotland, and there, on October 19, they boarded RMS *Cameronia* with nine hundred other passengers and headed to New York City. The ship had already made numerous round trips from Glasgow (and would make a total of eleven before being requisitioned as a troop ship). Moving in a convoy of three ships, the travel was slow and fraught with the fear that a torpedo from a German submarine would blow them out of the water. As it happened, the vessel in front of them hit a German mine and sank. Survivors were hauled aboard the *Cameronia*, the Hausners sharing their tiny cabin with two of them.[15]

But at least they were out of continental Europe, unlike Eisig's family members. They had chosen to remain in Poland and were not as fortunate. His brother Itzi and Itzi's son Fishel died in the Warsaw Ghetto. His brother Moshe was executed in the Ukrainian Borshchiv Ghetto, and his brother Mordko died somewhere in Russia.

At long last, in the morning hours of Monday, October 28, 1940, Helga, now four years old, was awakened by her mother, and the family went up to *Cameronia*'s deck. Under a brilliant blue sky, Mina told Helga, "I don't want you to ever forget what you're about to see."[16] The three watched in awe as they glided past the Statue of Liberty. After nearly a year in flight, having left everything behind and traveled more than 4,200 miles, the family had finally arrived in America. And they would begin their new life with new names. Eisig became

Ernst, Mina was now Mimi, and Helga adopted her more American-sounding middle name, Evelyn.

⟁

Three days after the *Cameronia* left Glasgow, eleven-year-old Rose Rehert became an orphan. By that time, her young life had already been fraught with drama and sorrow. Rose's father, Israel, had arrived in America from Russia in 1905. At seventeen, he had been sent from his home to avoid the czar's draft of uneducated Jewish boys. Settling in East Baltimore, a destination of many Russian Jews, Israel went to work in a sweatshop as a tailor.

Seven years later, Rose's mother, Fannie, arrived in East Baltimore from Lithuania with her older sister, Goldie. Fannie met and married Israel in 1917. Although she had come from a better economic background than Israel and arrived with more belongings, her health was frail. As a child she had contracted rheumatic fever, then a common inflammatory malady that followed a previous infection like strep throat. If the fever damaged heart valves, it became known as rheumatic heart disease. The symptoms of tender and extremely painful joints, chest pain, and fatigue subsided in mild cases. In severe cases, they persisted through the remainder of a patient's life. Fannie fell into the latter category.

Despite her frailty, she gave birth to sons Meyer, Paul, and Isaac (who became known as Ike) in the space of four years. The boys' memories of their mother varied, depending on the ebb and flow of Fannie's disease. They remembered the fainting spells, when Israel would revive her with spirits of ammonia, and the moans of pain only partially soothed with a hot water bottle.[17] Little Rose was born in 1929, seven years after Ike, and just four months before the stock market crash. Her memories of her mother were fewer, and always tinted by Fannie's worsening condition.[18]

When Rose was in first grade, Fannie suffered a stroke that paralyzed the right side of her body. Israel now had the responsibility of four children, plus juggling multiple jobs to keep food on the table. He was unable to provide much care to Fannie. So despite a cavalcade of housekeepers provided by the Associated Jewish Charities, her doctors decided it would be best for her to move into a "home for incurables." She was packed off to the Levindale Home for the Jewish Aged and Chronically Ill on Baltimore's Belvedere Avenue. Traveling an hour, via three different streetcars, Israel took Rose to visit every weekend until Fannie died there on January 29, 1939.

Months earlier, the family had already moved into Goldie's overcrowded home. In addition to Goldie's second husband, Harry, was her son from her first marriage, a large dog named Mottl, and a series of boarders who came and went as rooms were vacated. With the addition of five Reherts and a friend of Meyer's, the house was a noisy beehive, with little privacy.[19]

Rose had never learned English, speaking Yiddish with her parents her entire life to that point. That didn't change at Tante Goldie's. What did change was Israel. A year after Fannie died, he married Lottie Rubin, also a Russian immigrant, moving into her home five miles away. Everything Rose knew about stepmothers (primarily from fairy tales) could be boiled down to two words: *wicked* and *mean*. She simply refused to move with Israel, not wanting to leave behind the life that was familiar, albeit chaotic. It was probably just as well. In October 1940, a few short months after he married again, Israel died suddenly from a massive heart attack.

As the months passed, Tante Goldie's household began to shrink. Rose's eldest brother, Meyer, married and moved into his own apartment with his new wife. With the war roaring in Europe, brother Paul had joined the Merchant Marine. The youngest brother, Ike, with whom she was the closest, became the family's education pioneer, graduating from high school at sixteen and entering Western Maryland College on a full scholarship. This left Rose alone to deal with the family tyrant, Uncle Harry.

Harry Fischer was tall and balding, with a big belly and thick horn-rimmed glasses. He couldn't read or write a word of English but got a job at the post office nonetheless. He resented those who were smarter than he was, which was everyone in the family, including his wife. As Rose learned English and sailed from one grade to the next, Goldie tried in vain to stem her thirst for knowledge and quiet her desire to talk about all she was learning. Rose couldn't be silenced, however, a trait for which she would become famous. And the more she talked, the more verbally abusive Uncle Harry became toward her.

Rose was meticulous and motivated, and reading was a passion for her at Talmud Torah, the Board of Jewish Education school she attended until she was thirteen. Despite a brief suspension around the time of her father's second marriage, she excelled and moved on to Forest Park High School. Again, she stood out among her peers. But more important, the path to her future was becoming clearer.

Since Johns Hopkins Hospital was in the midst of her neighborhood, Rose had stared at its brick walls most of her life.[20] The idea of becoming a doctor was born early, growing stronger the older she got. On June 20, 1946, when she graduated from Forest Park, she stood at the threshold of making that dream a reality. She had received a Legislative Scholarship to the University of Maryland. But the $82 allotted annually for the first semester and the $83 available for the second didn't cover the entirety of the costs of attendance.

She next turned her sights on Johns Hopkins University. Although it didn't admit women at the time, she could attend its night school, McCoy College. But without a scholarship, she would need help. Harry and Goldie didn't have the money. Her brother Meyer had been working since he quit school at sixteen. He was the most likely to be financially able to loan her money. He was also of the common opinion that girls didn't need to go to college.[21] Clearly, it would be up to Rose to make a go of it on her own.

She enrolled, and despite cobbling together earnings from sales, secretarial, and sewing jobs, she couldn't come up with the $750 to cover the semester's tuition. Her account was marked as "delinquent," and she wasn't allowed to take the final exams. By year's end, she had traded in her school books for a job at an installment plan office. And that was when she met Dr. Horsley Gantt.

Dr. Gantt was the last student living outside of Russia who had been taught by the famed behavioral scientist Ivan Pavlov. Practicing psychiatry, Dr. Gantt ran the Hopkins Pavlovian Laboratory, using dogs just as his mentor had. He was struck by the self-assured eighteen-year-old Rose, whom he had met through a patient.

"Would you like to come work for me in the Pavlovian Lab?" he asked her. "The budget has been increased a little, but I'm afraid the job still can't pay you much."[22]

"Can I wear a white coat?" Rose asked.

"A what?"

"A white coat. The kind the medical students and interns wear."

"Of course. You've got to cover your clothing. You would work with dogs, and that can be messy."

"Say no more, Dr. Gantt. I've wanted to wear one of those white coats all my life."

The doctor was right about the pay. The salary of $130 a month (the equivalent of less than $2,000 today) wasn't much.[23] But Rose very much enjoyed her time in the lab. What she was absorbing from Dr. Gantt gave her a sense of accomplishment, along with a paycheck. She decided that she would save up her money and attend college once she had enough in the bank to cover at least the first few semesters. Something else, however, was weighing heavily on her mind.

When Rose's beloved brother Ike had graduated from Western Maryland College in 1942, he became the first Rehert with both high school and college degrees. Great things were expected of him. But life wasn't that simple. World War II was raging. Young American men were enlisting or being drafted for duty overseas at an astronomical rate. Ike had no stomach for war or killing. Consequently, he didn't register for the Selective Service, as he was legally bound to do, and was eventually arrested by the FBI.

Bailed out by a friend, Ike appeared for his trial a month later and pled not guilty, reading a sincere statement about his belief in brotherhood. War itself was the enemy the country needed to fight, he proclaimed. He was found guilty anyway and sentenced to three years in prison. Making the erroneous mental leap that education led to imprisonment, Rose's other brothers were even more determined to keep her out of college.

While Ike served his term, Rose kept up a steady stream of letters to him. They continued after he was released and went to Europe to work with a Quaker relief program. The postwar project took him from France to Italy and, ultimately, to Veldon, Austria, two hundred miles southeast of Vienna. He was shocked when in May 1949 a letter from Rose announced that she was coming to Europe to visit him. Dr. Gantt had given her a leave of absence until the end of October, and the savings from her rather meager earnings from the lab would make this dream trip possible.

Rose's Atlantic ship crossing was rather uneventful. It was the offseason for travel, since the universities were still in session.[24] Consequently, her traveling companions were mainly elderly couples. As luck would have it, she did meet an Indian gentleman from Bombay, who found her charming. He was traveling first class and invited her to join him on the upper deck each day. Rose found it as boring as tourist class, but at least she was bored in luxury during the seven-day trip. After arriving in Le Havre, France, she took a train to Paris and then another on to Austria.

Reuniting with Ike after three years was sheer joy. He took a week off from his own work, and after a tour of Vienna the two traveled by car to Genoa, Florence, and Venice. After that, they headed north to Germany, visiting the Kehlsteinhaus—Hitler's Eagle's Nest—and Munich. The trip's final destination was Dachau.

Only four years had passed since the Allies had entered the infamous concentration and extermination camp. Ike and Rose wandered through the crematorium and then entered the gas chamber. Standing side by side, they looked up at the round circle in the ceiling from which the Nazis had intended to drop gas pellets as they did in so many other camps, murdering hundreds of thousands of Jews. The moment was chilling, too poignant for words. Rose would later say that although she had lived her entire life in a Jewish home, she had never felt her Jewishness so keenly.[25]

She stayed with Ike in Austria for a few more weeks before striking out on her own. Postcards from Switzerland, Luxembourg, Belgium, the Netherlands, and Paris kept him apprised of her adventures. In mid-October, Rose called him to say she was ready to go home. While she would have preferred to travel by ship, she told him she couldn't find passage. So she had booked an overnight Air France flight from Paris to New York. The flight would leave at 8:00 p.m. on

October 27, with a short refueling stop on the Portuguese island of Santa Maria, in the Azores, before flying on to the United States.

Ike, however, thought Rose deserved another adventure by sea. He told a British friend in Austria about her inability to find space aboard a ship, knowing that the friend had a buddy in the travel agency business. Ike's friend made a call to his buddy's office on Ike's behalf, and a ticket aboard the SS *Washington* was procured. So Rose canceled her flight, leaving instead from Southampton on Friday, October 28, and arriving in New York City on November 4.

Once back in the States, Rose was shocked at the horrific news that the flight she had been scheduled to take, Air France flight 009, had disappeared. The plane had left Paris's Orly Airport at 8:05 p.m. There were thirty-seven passengers on board, with eleven crew members. At 2:51 the next morning, October 28, the pilot radioed the Santa Maria airport. The Lockheed Constellation was at a height of 3,000 feet, he reported, and they had the airport in sight. Then the radio went silent.[26]

Receiving no response to its calls, the airport tower dispatched a search involving eight aircraft and a number of ships. Rescuers finally spotted what was left of the plane on the side of Pico Redondo, a mountain on the nearby island of São Miguel. It was sixty miles off course from where it should have been. They found wreckage spread over five hundred square yards, and the bodies of all forty-eight souls who had been on board. Fate had seen fit to keep Rose from being one of them.

⁓

It is not uncommon in the course of a human life that injury, disaster, and death are inexplicably avoided. And often those near misses go completely unrecognized by the individual. Shirley, Evelyn, and Rose had most likely never heard of Mary Cassatt's prediction to Theodate Pope. Yet they were clearly remarkable examples of being saved for "something else," for without them, the lives of millions of women would have played out very differently.

Chapter 2

~

I Know Quite as Much as I Need To

In 1950, the Hausners' apartment on West 86th Street was an epicenter of activity. It was their third home in New York City. The first had been a temporary shelter on the Lower East Side, situated near the docks; numerous such shelters were run by charitable organizations, and they often were a first stop for Jewish immigrants. Newcomers, like the Hausners, could stay for three or four weeks, free of charge, to find employment and a more permanent address. The next move took the family to Columbus Avenue, on the Upper West Side. Eventually they finally settled a few blocks away, on 86th Street.

It has been said that the real heroes of the immigrant wave during the 1940s were the women, many of whom came from middle- to upper-class backgrounds, as Mimi had.[1] They were accustomed to decorating their homes with fine furnishings and buying nice clothing for themselves and their families. They longed to live similarly in America, and that goal gave them the impetus to seek ways to earn money, even though they didn't necessarily have previous experience or sufficient education. They became shopgirls or bakery clerks, governesses or kindergarten aides. Some even went door-to-door selling the new Avon cosmetics. Rather than equating work with a loss of dignity, they saw it as a faster road to get back to their previous ways of life.

Since Mimi had been Ernst's hat designer in Vienna, following a similar path came naturally. And by this time her parents had arrived from Austria, as had her sister and brother-in-law. Surviving members of Ernst's family had immigrated, too, although the absence of his three brothers and a nephew left a void at Sabbath meals. But as newly naturalized Americans, Ernst and Mimi always aimed their gaze forward.

Little Evelyn had figured that out for herself. She had realized shortly after their arrival that Germany and Germans were the enemy during the war years, and her mind absorbed the English language like a sponge. By the time she entered school, she was nearly fluent. Meanwhile, Mimi and Ernst's basic knowledge of the language had improved so much that by 1947 they had become the proud owners of the Lamay Dress Shop. Ernst was once again in his element, charming his female customers with his European flair.[2]

And his business plan was ingenious. Each year, he would buy the previous season's dress inventory (at discount prices, of course) and hold it until the following year. He would then sell those items to women who sought out the "latest" designs. With the example of her parents' courage and ingenuity, it was no surprise that Evelyn would use retail sales as a way to advance herself. But first, she would get an education.

As the 1940s became the 1950s, America existed in a tense "watch and wait" state. The United States had been the first to develop and use atomic bombs, but it wouldn't be long before a weapon of that power would be created by others as well. Meanwhile, the Soviet Union and China were keen to expand their brands of communism to neighboring countries. A common idea at the time was that the single most important way to preserve America was to preserve what was assumed to make it superior to and different from the communist countries: the nuclear family. And that, it was thought, could be done only if women remained in their proper role as homemakers.[3]

The good news was that the U.S. marriage rate had risen to an all-time high, with the number of women tying the knot right out of high school climbing, too. And even many of those who did enter college were there only to earn their "M.R.S. degree"—the one that came not with a diploma but a ring on the third finger of the left hand. Consequently, women typically either didn't complete college or married soon after finishing. University enrollments in 1954 favored men nine to one. Of the 2,653,034 students enrolled that year, 26,530 were women. That number included Evelyn Hausner, who had enrolled in Hunter College that fall.[4]

Hunter's origins stem back to the nineteenth-century "normal school" movement, which educated women to become teachers. At the end of the century, the Normal College of the City of New York changed its name to honor its founder, Thomas Hunter. Snuggled between Park and Lexington Avenues at 68th Street, the school had built a reputation for developing smart and savvy women. That appealed to Evelyn, as did the fact that Hunter, as a part of the city's university system, was free for New Yorkers.

Evelyn bought into the idea of the "M.R.S. degree," and so her plan was to meet and marry a lawyer.[5] Since Hunter was a women's college, she needed to expand her search territory. The venerable Barnes and Noble bookstore on Fifth Avenue at 18th Street provided the perfect hunting ground. "The book corner of the world" (as B&N billed itself) was located just a few blocks from New York University's law school. The store had launched a campaign encouraging students to sell back their used textbooks for cash.[6] The bookstore's hope was that they would use that cash to buy used books for the next term, while the store resold their old books to other students. And law students needed lots of books. Evelyn began working at Barnes and Noble over winter break, remembering in her memoir, "It paid $5 an hour, which was a lot for 1955. I was earning $40 a day!" ($460 in today's money).[7]

Not long after Evelyn started her job, her high school chum Stephanie Fishman called her. "She had met a great fellow down in Florida over the Christmas break," Evelyn explained. "His name was Bob Nishball and he was in New York with his best friend, Leonard Lauder. Would I like to come to her house on Friday for a party her parents were giving for their friends?" Evelyn agreed, and thought the "well-dressed, smart, poised young man" who came to pick her up was also smart, as he chatted respectfully with Ernst.[8]

After the party, Leonard took Evelyn home in a taxi and gave her a goodnight peck on the cheek. When she opened the door to her parents' second-floor apartment, she found her father waiting for her, and she panicked. He'd never waited up for her before; had something happened to her mother? Ernst reassured her: "She's okay. I just wanted you to know that that's a nice boy."

Leonard Lauder wasn't a lawyer, but he was indeed a nice boy. He was the eldest son of Joe Lauder and the soon-to-be-famous Estée Lauder. Like the Hausners, Josephine Esther Mentzer's parents had immigrated from Eastern Europe in the first decade of the twentieth century. Unlike the Hausners, they weren't fleeing certain persecution and potential death; they came to make a better life for themselves. Josephine's family had nicknamed her "Esty," which she fashioned into the more exotic "Estée."

Estée's uncle John Schotz was a chemist who also had immigrated to America. In 1923, he launched New Way Laboratories, where he produced Flory Anna Eczema Ointment, named for his wife.[9] The concoction addressed more than just eczema. Its advertisements claimed it also tackled pimples, burns, cracked hands, ringworm, and piles (the era's term for hemorrhoids). But Uncle John was developing other creams, too, including one that enraptured young Estée. It was velvety, smelled divine, and had a nearly magical transformative effect on the skin.

After her marriage to Joseph Lauter in 1930 (she would soon reimagine their last name as Lauder), she repackaged Uncle John's cream, calling it Super Rich All-Purpose Cream. Under the company name Lauter Associates Chemists, she set up concessions in beauty salons. Estée was fearless at giving demonstrations and passing out samples, two revolutionary sales tactics she would become known for. After Leonard was born in 1933, she began taking him on her sales trips to Miami, where rich women gathered in the winter. Chatting up potential customers as she sauntered through resorts and around the swimming pools, she soon had a loyal, albeit small, clientele.[10]

At thirteen, Leonard began working as a paid employee, first in the plant, then typing invoices, and then moving into more responsible positions before going to the University of Pennsylvania. He had joined the Navy after his 1954 graduation and was about to begin its Officer Candidate School. And then came that blind date with Evelyn, whom he found very attractive. "She laughed a lot," he wrote in his autobiography, "but in a natural way, not at all forced. . . . I was definitely interested in Evelyn from that moment."[11]

They continued dating throughout his time at Officer Candidate School and then during his stint at the Navy's Supply School. When he went to sea they wrote each other as well. It all made Estée happy. "You know," she told Leonard, "of all the girls you've gone out with, the only one I really like is Evelyn."[12]

Estée wasn't alone in her affection for Evelyn. After Evelyn graduated from Hunter in June 1958, she put her degree to use, teaching at an all-Black elementary school in Harlem. Her shadowy childhood memories of escape and the way she'd grown up as an outsider might have been her impetus to motivate disadvantaged students toward success. But the school's fifth and sixth graders initially weren't sure what to make of the petite white woman. "They tested me every single day," Evelyn recalled. "But I established my authority, and earned their respect."[13] And the students loved her.

Across town, and with the Navy behind him, Leonard joined the company full-time. In December, he invited Evelyn to his family's Palm Beach house for New Year's. Midway through the vacation, Joe and Estée had to go back to New York suddenly, leaving the couple alone without a proper chaperone. Leonard said to her, "Now I *have* to marry you."

"Is that a proposal?" she asked.

He told her it was.[14]

On July 5, 1959, Evelyn became Mrs. Leonard Lauder in an evening ceremony at New York's Plaza Hotel. Bob Nishball was Leonard's best man, completing the circle, since it was because of Bob and his date Stephanie that the newlyweds had met. They honeymooned in Banff, Alberta, then flew to San Francisco. Leonard had visited California many times, but it was Evelyn's first trip. They saw everything required of tourists before they flew on to Los Angeles.

The grand opening of the brand-new Estée Lauder beauty counter at Bullocks Wilshire—the most elegant store in the city—was happening while they were there. Leonard had had a brilliant marketing idea: a specially designed petite powder compact, an innovation over the larger ones traditionally sold. The company was giving them away for free, just for stopping by the counter. Of course, the hope was that the women would also buy products.

Leonard and Evelyn were shocked to see a line of women snaking far up Wilshire Boulevard, waiting for the doors to open. His idea had certainly worked. Moreover, news about the storm of customers on Wilshire spread to the Bullocks stores in Santa Ana and Pasadena. Leonard and Evelyn traveled to both those locations, too, leaving each with an agreement to carry Estée Lauder cosmetics, beginning with the compact giveaway.

Back on home turf in Manhattan, the young couple settled into a cozy one-bedroom apartment on East 63rd Street. It was like a little dollhouse, with a kitchen, one bedroom, one bathroom, and a living room with a dining alcove. Leonard went back to work, although the company was so small he didn't have his own office or even a proper title. And although Evelyn had loved teaching, after just one year she gave it up. In that era, German measles was prevalent among school-age children. With a vaccine not yet created, it was a dangerous disease for a pregnant woman. And Mrs. Lauder was pregnant.

⟶

The scene is the middle of the night, early 1920s. In the upper hallway of Downton Abbey, a cluster of men—Lord Grantham, Matthew Crowley, and Tom Branson (the expectant father)—anxiously await news from the pregnant Lady Sybil's bedchamber. When Dr. Clarkson, the family's physician, emerges with Lady Grantham and Sybil's sisters, he announces to the men, "Everything's fine."[15]

"You mean it was a false alarm?" Lord Grantham asks.

"Not exactly," the good doctor begins to explain. "These early labor pains show that the womb is preparing itself for—"

At the word *womb*, Lord Grantham uncomfortably drops his eyes, as if Clarkson had just, well, said the word *womb*.

In reverse patronization for the time, Lady Grantham interrupts Clarkson. "I'm afraid that Lord Grantham doesn't enjoy medical detail." And the conversation comes to a close.

Over the course of history, women's health discussions have centered solely on the very organ that made Lord Grantham blush: the womb, aka the uterus. In the fifth century BC, the Greek physician Hippocrates proclaimed that nearly all of a woman's physical and psychological problems stemmed from a migratory uterus. His explanation was that the uterus (*hysteron* in Greek) literally roamed throughout the entirety of a woman's body, provoking illness and disruption wherever it briefly came to rest before moving on to other parts of the body.[16] The resulting condition, which Hippocrates called *hysteria,* soon became a catch-all for anything about women men couldn't identify or weren't happy about, including women exerting their independence. Control the uterus, the thinking went, and the woman could be controlled as well.

As time marched forward, a variety of prescriptions were heralded for the wandering womb. Pungent scents were placed under a woman's nose if the uterus was thought to have moved to her upper body; pleasant-smelling ones were laid near the vagina to coax the *hysteron* back south. Marriage and sex were highly recommended for hysteria, while masturbating would surely exacerbate the condition. In the nineteenth century, the ultimate cure for hysteria was locking the woman up, along with her evil uterus. This was very convenient: doctors were better able to study their patients, fathers could force daughters to conform, and husbands could do the same, along with carrying on affairs.[17]

The disgraceful truth is that many of the women who were deemed hysterical actually suffered from what we now know are mental or neurological illnesses. Since disproportionately more women than men were assumed to be suffering from schizophrenia, depression, borderline personality disorder, anxiety, epilepsy, and more (all of which fell into the hysteria bucket), it was a tidy diagnosis. The venerable Sigmund Freud described hysteria as "characteristically feminine." This non-disorder did not disappear from the American Psychiatric Association's bible of modern psychiatry, the *Diagnostic and Statistical Manual of Mental Disorders,* until 1980.[18]

Even after the retirement of hysteria as a condition, menstruation, pregnancy, and menopause—and the hormones controlling them—remained a messy mystery both to male physicians and to the male population at large. Returning to Downton Abbey: Dr. Clarkson is once again visiting. This time, he and Lord Grantham are sipping whiskey in the library, discussing Lady Grantham's surprise pregnancy.[19]

"It's unusual, obviously," Dr. Clarkson observes.

"Unusual? It's biblical!" Lord Grantham proclaims.

"Not quite. You understand that women go through a certain change. . . ."

Lord Grantham waves his hand, as if batting away the words. "Thank you. I know quite as much as I need to about all that." He follows that discussion-ending statement with a large gulp of whiskey.

If medicine, and society at large, had little interest in understanding the part of a woman's body responsible for reproduction, the same was true for a woman's breasts. They fed children and were fun to fondle. Period. The idea of breast health, breast irregularities, and breast cancer would not be a part of any medical school curriculum for a very, very long time. Understanding that blatant lack of interest in the health of half of the population is critical to understanding why the women's health movement and the breast cancer movement were so significant.

Nor was the controlling part of the population interested in training women to care for other women. The difference in the genders was thought to imply an inferior mental capacity in the fairer sex; it prevented them from being able to participate in politics or voting, and from comprehending anything that was taught in higher education.

That was precisely the slant of the address Dr. Edward Hammond Clarke delivered to the New England Women's Club on December 14, 1872. The chill in the Boston air that Saturday morning matched the understandable reception the Harvard Medical School professor received from his audience. Too much education, he said, would divert women from their "divinely-appointed field of operation" (i.e., as baby factories) and render them "weak, neuralgic, dyspeptic, [and] hysterical." It was a position he espoused until his death three years later of "intestinal" (probably colon) cancer, a disease against which many twenty-first-century women researchers would go on to make great strides.

Baltimore Junior College had been founded in 1947 to provide post-high-school education to the city's World War II veterans. By 1950, the school had an enrollment of 431 students, Rose Rehert among them.[20] She had never abandoned the idea of a college degree, determined to earn it no matter how many tiny steps she had to take, squeezing in night classes around her job with Dr. Gantt. She wasn't even slowed down by her appendectomy in November of that year. Rose spent her four-week recovery working madly on assignments from her hospital bed and then back home at Goldie's. When the semester ended in early December, she received a grade of excellent and accolades from the dean.[21]

Remarkably, that wasn't the highlight of the month. Rose had a friend, Alex Martick, whose parents owned the Tyson Street Tavern in downtown Baltimore.[22] Playing the part of matchmaker, Alex thought she'd be perfect for another friend of his, Harvey Kushner, and he set up a time for them to meet at the tavern. Given that the place became a gay bar at night, it didn't dawn on Rose or Harvey that Alex had romance in mind. In fact, each of them assumed the other was gay, and that well-meaning Alex was just introducing them to be friends. Sitting in a dark corner of the knotty-pine-paneled bar, under the fake Tiffany lights, they soon surmised the truth. And Alex scored a ten in matchmaking: it didn't take long for Rose and Harvey to fall in love.

Harvey would be graduating from Johns Hopkins with an engineering degree the following June. Insomuch as the Korean War had begun six months earlier, he said to Rose a few weeks later, "Are we gonna get married? Because if we're not, I'll be going to Korea as soon as I'm out of college."[23] An engagement announcement appeared in the newspaper in January 1951. But Rose had already begun courting another love: journalism.

There was something about weaving together a story that appealed to her. And she had a wonderful knack for it. That knack had garnered her the position of feature editor of *The Crier*, Baltimore Junior College's newspaper. The more she was exposed to writing, the better writer she became. She greatly impressed the faculty advisor and was selected to be one of the two delegates to attend the annual convention of the prestigious Columbia Scholastic Press Association.

The Columbia University event, occurring in March in New York City, was considered the pinnacle of a scholastic journalist's career. It was attended by newspaper staffs from around the country, and it kicked off with a dinner at the Men's Faculty Club. Following that the next day were forums and clinics, along with a tour of Gotham. The conference wrapped up with a grand luncheon at the Waldorf-Astoria Hotel, where the young journalists were treated to a swank meal and speeches from key luminaries in collegiate publishing.

Soon after she returned to Baltimore, Rose and Harvey were married. In fact, they were married twice in the spring of 1951. The first was in the office of a justice of the peace, and the second was in a more traditional Jewish ceremony to appease Goldie and others in the family. When their first baby was born less than nine months after the Jewish service, tongues wagged. But Rose and Harvey didn't care: their son was perfect. She had wanted to honor her dear friend Dr. Horsley Gantt by naming her son after him. But she couldn't bring herself to saddle a child with such an out-of-fashion first name. So they settled on the doctor's last name as the baby's first name.

Two and a half years later, Gantt was joined by little brother Stephen. But the joy the Kushners had experienced earlier was not to be repeated. Stephen had a birth defect, suffering from a congenital malformation of his heart valves. While the condition might be repairable today, it was not in 1954, and he died at just three weeks old. The experience was difficult for the young parents, but years later Rose would draw on that grief.

And the Kushner family continued to grow. Todd arrived in 1956, and she and Harvey welcomed daughter Lesley in 1958. Mothering three children under the age of seven was a full-time job, causing Rose to pause both her education and her writing. But her interest in them never waned. When her brother Ike became the family's first duly employed journalist, signing on with the *Baltimore Sun* in 1960, Rose was both proud of him and thrilled at the thought that her brother's employment meant a possible foot in the newspaper's door for her.

～

The always-sunny Shirley Temple had had plenty of experience with newspapers in her short life. As a movie star, of course, she knew their value in promoting a film and an actor. Shirley hoped the press coverage of her work during World War II, as she traveled to USO shows and visited wounded veterans in hospitals after they returned to the United States, would inspire readers to do whatever they could for the war effort. But eager reporters also sought out any inkling of romance in the young woman's life.

Despite her fame and fortune, Shirley's goal for the future had always been to become a wife and a mother. At fifteen, she announced that she would marry at seventeen.[24] To that end, she looked at every boy she met as potential husband material. And she measured each against five non-negotiable qualities: he couldn't be in the movies; he had to be at least five years older than she was; he had to be handsome; he had to be smart; and, most important, he had to be completely nonplussed by her fame. If the young man had never seen *any* of her films, all the better. John Agar Jr. would fit that bill.

On a lovely summer day in 1943, Shirley went to a swim party given by the daughter of her Beverly Hills neighbor, actress ZaSu Pitts. Also on the guest list was Joyce Agar, whom Shirley knew from the Westlake School for Girls, where both were students. Joyce brought along her big brother, Jack (as John was known). Twenty-three and home on leave from the Army Air Corps, Jack barely remembered that fifteen-year-old Shirley had been in movies. Tall, athletic, and handsome, Jack was completely disinterested in her star power. Without breaking a sweat, he had met nearly every requirement on her list, and she was smitten.

When the fall term began, Shirley's older classmates at Westlake were writing to their boyfriends who were serving in the military. So she wrote to Jack, and he responded. Several letters—and months—later, he told her would be home for the 1944 Christmas holiday on a ten-day furlough. He was surprised by the girl who was waiting for him, now a year older. She was much more sophisticated than the other girls he had dated. By the end of those ten days, Jack and Shirley had fallen in love.

As 1945 dawned, newspapers filled their pages with the dramatic events unfolding in both the European and Pacific theaters of World War II. The young couple figured it was just a matter of time before he'd be shipped off. Now stationed near Spokane, he came to Los Angeles on a three-day pass the first week of April. Sitting in a car on Sunset Boulevard, under a clear night sky, Jack produced an engagement ring, and Shirley said yes.

The Temples liked Jack and were satisfied with the engagement, as long as the couple would wait until Shirley was eighteen to marry. That was a year away. As soon as she graduated from Westlake in June 1945, she persuaded them to allow her to marry Jack in the fall. They ultimately agreed, and the wedding planning went into full swing.

"Shirley Temple today began what she considers the greatest role of her life—that of Mrs. John Agar," the Associated Press said of the September 19 event.[25] Shirley had been determined not to "make a circus" of her wedding, but the twelve thousand fans gathered outside the Wilshire Methodist Church had other plans, cheering madly when the newly married couple came out the front door.

Ready to reenter Hollywood, Shirley sought roles more aligned with her age. It wasn't long before cracks began to appear in the marriage. Jack was not of the temperament to be "Mr. Shirley Temple," and Shirley didn't want him to be. Unfortunately, however, the couple needed a movie star's salary to live in the comfortable fashion they had envisioned. The answer to the dilemma was for Jack to become an actor as well and build his own career.

"He's a natural," Shirley said of her tall and handsome husband. "That's why I married him. That, and a couple of other reasons, too."[26] Jack was under contract, as Shirley was, with David O. Selznick's studio. In June 1947, they were cast together in director John Ford's star-packed film *War Party*. Jack would play the part of an Indian scout, so he had to learn to ride a horse bareback for his role. Just as shooting began a month later, big news broke on the set. Director Ford was changing the movie's title to *Fort Apache*. And Shirley, who was cast in the part of the daughter of the fort's newly arrived commander (played by Henry Fonda), was five months pregnant.

Jack was thrilled at the prospect of fatherhood and by his first acting job. Plus he'd found a new friend. Veteran actor John Wayne, fourteen years older than Jack, took his young co-star under his wing. Jack had already been drinking heavily every night. Now it was accelerated by the equally bibulous Wayne. Jack began staying out late, a pattern that continued throughout the rest of Shirley's pregnancy. When labor began at three o'clock the morning of January 30, 1948 (which happened to be Jack's birthday), she couldn't rouse him from an alcohol-induced sleep. She drove herself to the hospital, and a few hours later their daughter Linda Susan (who would be known by her middle name) was born.

Jack was inspired to give up booze for a while, but his abstinence was short-lived. Another year of drinking, womanizing, and fighting was all Shirley could take. Returning to California from Harry Truman's presidential inauguration in January 1949, she hired a law firm to, as she put it, "terminate a marriage that has already ended."[27]

The final paperwork was signed on December 5, 1949, stating that Shirley had full custody of Linda Susan. She would take back her maiden name, and Jack would receive half of her earnings from 1945 to the date of the decree, part of which would go into a trust for their daughter. With remarkable prescience, just a few months after their marriage Shirley's father had had Jack sign a quit-claim deed, confirming that all of Shirley's premarital property belonged solely to her.

Ready to move into the new decade with a clean slate, Shirley could think of no better place to begin than in Hawaii. Off they flew to Honolulu—Shirley, her parents, Susan (who would celebrate her second birthday on the island), and a nanny—staying first at the luxurious Royal Hawaiian Hotel, and then renting a lovely little house in the quiet residential enclave of Kahala.

A week after their arrival, Hawaiian real estate titan Earl Thacker and his wife hosted an afternoon cocktail party for them at their Diamond Head home. One of the invited guests, an avid surfer, told the hosts he would attend only if the waves weren't up. Fortunately for Shirley, it was a relatively calm day on the Pacific Ocean.

"Charlie Black," the tall, tanned, handsome man said, sticking out his hand to shake. "You're new here. Somebody's secretary?"[28] His genuine ignorance of who Shirley was became just one of the characteristics Shirley found endearing about Charlie. They spent an hour chatting about their lives, their interests, and their families, and then set up a date to drive around the island of Oahu. The next day he arrived toting a skiff and took her out to swim around a favorite reef.

Charlie never touched his surfboard after that first handshake. Twelve days later, they agreed that since each of their lives was going nowhere, they might as well go together. This time, however, Shirley put several safety nets in place to make certain her heart wouldn't be broken again.

She returned to California on March 12. While their love letters crisscrossed the Pacific, Shirley activated the first of those nets. She called FBI director J. Edgar Hoover, still a family friend more than a decade after the *Blue Bird* incident. Just who was Charles Alden Black? she wanted to know. She had already decided that if he was anything other than what he had represented, the relationship would be over immediately. Hoover was happy to help. When a local agent came to her home a few weeks later to give her a report, she sighed with relief. Charlie was exactly who he said he was: the son of a San Franciso businessman, a graduate of Harvard, a former mariner with the Merchant Marine, and a naval PT boat captain during World War II. Currently, just as Charlie had told her, he was working for the Hawaiian Pineapple Company.

By this time, the two were overwhelmed with loneliness and their desire to be together. In early summer, as they had planned, Charlie quit his job and came to California. Once he arrived in Los Angeles, discretion was going to be crucial. Shirley's divorce was interlocutory, meaning that if something occurred during the first year that suggested she was an unfit mother, Susan could be removed from her custody. Being seen snuggling up to a new man would certainly raise eyebrows.

Consequently, Charlie became known as a houseguest of Shirley's parents. If they were seen in public, he was introduced as a family friend. They all lived in quiet seclusion behind the secure walls of their Beverly Hills estate. Those five months gave Shirley ample time to discover any major flaws in Charlie *before* they became husband and wife. It was Shirley's second safety net.

On December 6, 1950, Shirley's divorce became absolute, with all restrictions removed. Ten days later, she and Charlie were married at his parents' beautiful summer home in Del Monte, just east of Monterey. The Mission-style home was the perfect setting for the family-only ceremony. With the high-beamed ceiling, the fireplace mantel festooned with pine boughs and flowers, and a cheerful fire warming the chill air, they exchanged vows. The new couple honeymooned in Pebble Beach for several days before heading to the Black family home in San Francisco. Ever the dutiful star, Shirley held a press conference to introduce her new husband. But that wasn't the only story she gave the assembled reporters.

"I have signed a new contract with Charles," she explained, "the only contract I have."[29] At twenty-two, she had been in films for nineteen years. She was the most popular movie star in America between 1935 and 1939 (even more popular than Clark Gable) and had been photographed more frequently than President Franklin Roosevelt. But now, she told the world, she was officially retired. Her only roles were as wife and mother.

Six months earlier, the Chinese-backed North Koreans had invaded South Korea, launching the peninsula into war. As a commander in the Navy Reserve, Charlie was ordered to report for duty in Washington, D.C., in April 1951. So he, Shirley, and Susan embarked on a cross-country road trip. The second day, they stopped for lunch in Prague, Oklahoma, named for the hometown of its Czech settlers. When they arrived at the Will Rogers Hotel for the night, Shirley suddenly experienced severe abdominal pains. Charlie took her immediately to the hospital, where she underwent an emergency appendectomy.

As she came to in her hospital room, her husband's face loomed above her, holding up a jar containing her appendix. The little pink finger-shaped organ, floating around in liquid, looked perfectly benign. It had none of the deadly features she'd assumed she would see, given the surgeon's warning of the risk if she hesitated to have it removed.

"Doc says it's the most perfect appendix he's ever seen," Charlie told her. Shirley was confused. Why the reversal of opinion? Charlie explained. "The tune changed after the operation, when he began singing that he took it out to be on the safe side."[30] Shirley's pain, he continued, was probably food poisoning, a gift from the ham sandwich she'd eaten in Prague. What a debacle. The unnecessary surgery had completely derailed their plans for a family trip. Now Charlie would have to go on to D.C. alone to honor his report date. Shirley and Susan would follow when she was able to travel. But it was a medical lesson: no matter the urgency, ask adequate questions and understand the answers before undergoing surgery. This would serve her well in the future.

Chapter 3

⁓

Remember the Ladies

"We stand today on the edge of a new frontier—the frontier of the 1960s—a frontier of unknown opportunities and perils, a frontier of unfulfilled hopes and threats."[1] As John Fitzgerald Kennedy accepted the nomination for president, his twenty-one-minute speech at the 1960 Democratic convention was replete with exciting challenges. And the sixty thousand Americans who nearly filled the Los Angeles Memorial Coliseum erupted into resounding applause at every opportunity.[2]

"But I tell you the new frontier is here, whether we seek it or not," the newly minted candidate continued. "Beyond that frontier are uncharted areas of science and space, unsolved problems of peace and war. . . . It would be easier to shrink back from that frontier. . . . But I believe the times demand invention, innovation, imagination, decision. I am asking each of you to be new pioneers on that new frontier."

President Franklin Roosevelt was sixty-three years old when he died in office. His successor, Harry Truman, was sixty-nine the day he turned over the presidential reins to Dwight Eisenhower, who, at seventy-one, would now be leaving the job. A new frontier, led by this vigorous, handsome young man, just forty-three years old, and his beautiful, glamorous wife (a mere thirty-one), promised something the country had never seen. For half of America, however, that new frontier wouldn't embody much change from the old one.

In 1960, there were 91,128,169 women in the United States, making up 50.44 percent of the population.[3] One in ten of those was head of her household.[4] But no matter their job, working women made only three-fifths the wages men earned. Fewer than 5 percent of them had a college degree. Only 2 percent of medical school students were women, with female doctors making up just 5 percent of the profession.[5] The two women senators in Washington, D.C., and their seventeen sisters in the House equated to 2 and 3.9 percent of their chambers' totals, respectively.[6] These numbers clearly reflected the continuing opinion that a woman's place was in the home.

At the same time in Congress, there were over four hundred pieces of legislation that would affect women, languishing unpassed in various stages. Most of them included "protective" labor laws, created to ensure that women were placed in "appropriate" positions for their gender, most often with regard to their strength level and what they were able to accomplish in a dress. Expressed another way, those laws urged that, due to women's biological differences, workplace accommodations for them were required. Employers (via their senators and representatives) pushed back on those complications and simply continued hiring men. And then an interesting thing happened.

A large part of Kennedy's presidential victory was due to women. Those in his family and extended family recruited other women, who in turn recruited more, including the Women's Committee of the International Confederation of Free Trade Unions. Together, they all delivered the votes Kennedy needed in his extremely close win. The female election army's long-sought reward came on December 14, 1961, with Kennedy's creation of the Presidential Commission on the Status of Women. The twenty-eight-member commission would be headed by former First Lady Eleanor Roosevelt.

In a televised 1962 discussion with Mrs. Roosevelt, Kennedy said, "We want to be sure that women are used as effectively as they can be to provide a better life for our people, in addition to meeting their primary responsibility, which is in the home."[7] The latter part of that statement was a foreshadowing of what was to come.

When the commission presented its final report on October 11, 1963 (just six weeks before the president's assassination), it wasn't what Kennedy's female army had hoped for. The statement spoke of the inequalities facing women, while still acknowledging their traditional gender-specific roles as wife, mother, and homemaker.

Disappointingly, the summary noted that women were already given equal rights under the Fourteenth Amendment of the Constitution, and they were supposed to be protected against being deprived of life, liberty, and property, also provided for by the Constitution. There was no need for further amendments, the report concluded.[8] After all, thanks to the first wave of feminism at the turn of the twentieth century, women already had the most precious right: they could vote.

As in earlier decades, many women felt as though their needs weren't being met, and the report's summation didn't do much to assuage those feelings. The commission laid out three major steps the president should put into motion immediately, beginning with, once again, encouraging private employers to treat women equally. Second, the commission felt Kennedy should designate a cabinet member to make certain their recommendations were being followed. And finally, the commission members felt a federal program for women's education was needed, because, the report stated, they "can look forward to a number of useful years after raising families."

Evelyn and Leonard's first son, William, was born in 1960, followed by his brother, Gary, two years later. But Evelyn had no intention of waiting until after her children were raised in order to be "useful." She came from a family of industrious men *and* women. And while her decision not to return to her Harlem classroom in the fall of 1959 had been disappointing to her, Leonard softened that disappointment by suggesting she work in the family business. He had no doubt she'd be successful; he had already seen her in action a few years before.

Shortly after he had proposed and upon their return to New York from Palm Beach, Evelyn had joined him on a visit to the city's iconic department store Bloomingdale's, on Lexington Avenue. Leonard needed to have a quick meeting with the beauty consultant at the Estée Lauder counter and asked Evelyn if she would mind keeping an eye on the counter while he took the consultant out for a cup of coffee. When the two returned, there was such a crowd in front of the counter, Leonard couldn't even see his fiancée. Weaving through the excited women, he spotted her in the center of the action, busily selling products.

Evelyn's observations of her parents in their Vienna and New York stores, combined with her education as a teacher, gave her a unique skill set. She became a jack-of-all-trades at Estée Lauder, filling in behind counters, handling quality control, and, most creatively, as the company receptionist. She would answer the phone with a German accent, then "transfer" the call to the correct department, only to return to the line as another employee, minus the accent.[9] As time went on, Evelyn's contribution to the company grew. She became "Miss Evelyn, Estée Lauder's famous beauty consultant," traveling from store to store. She showed customers how to be "more radiant and beautiful" with the company's products. From that position, she launched training schools, teaching the company's beauty advisors how to do what she did.

Perhaps Evelyn's most unique title was that of guinea pig. "I'm a liaison between my mother-in-law who creates new products, and my husband who, as executive vice president, sells them," she explained to a reporter. "They try out everything on me. Sometimes just for my opinion, but usually literally."[10]

For her part, Estée adored Evelyn, feeling she was a huge asset to the company. In fact, Estée often referred to Evelyn as "the daughter she never had."[11] Both women had strong personalities, but Evelyn was one of the few people who spoke her mind to Estée. She attributed that frankness to her childhood, having had to fend for herself as an immigrant child in a new country. The women's relationship was truly tested when Leonard proposed the creation of an entirely new line for the company.

Stepping out of the corporate comfort zone was not the new part. Following Chanel and Fabergé, he had created and launched Lauder's men's line, Estée Lauder's Aramis, in time for the 1963 holiday season. But, as Leonard told Evelyn, he had begun to notice the increasing use of the word *hypoallergenic* in cosmetic ads. What if Estée Lauder became the first premium makeup brand that offered a line in that category?

They tapped the most famous dermatologist in New York City, who would develop the formulas for the new line. Next, they pursued (and hired) *Vogue* magazine's beauty editor to conceptualize the marketing campaign. She came up with the famous countertop "computer" that analyzed a woman's skin via some basic questions. But what would they call this new line?

On a trip to Paris in the midst of the line's development, Evelyn saw a sign reading *Clinique Esthétique.* She translated it for Leonard: Aesthetics Clinic. The phrase conveyed precisely that the salon's specialty was skincare.[12] The simple word *clinique* was perfect for their new skincare line, giving it a "doctor-approved" feel. Estée, however, was not a fan. She had never sold a product that didn't carry her name, and she wasn't keen to start. She was even slower to embrace Evelyn's idea that the Clinique saleswomen wear white lab coats. Estée said they looked like doctors, which Evelyn told her was the point. Despite Estée's concerns, the success of the September 9, 1968, Clinique launch was earth-shattering.

But Evelyn knew there was still a great deal she could learn from Estée, and she was eager to do so. When the company received a fresh volley of cosmetic challenges from Revlon (founded and led by Charles Revson), Estée was quick to point out that because she was a woman, she knew what women wanted in their makeup. On the other hand, Charles Revson "made every model [in his ads] look like a mistress because he thought every woman wanted to *be* a mistress."[13]

As the company expanded outside America's borders, Estée made another cogent observation: "In many ways women share a common language. No matter what our culture, no matter what our background, we understand each other."[14]

Those two notions—that men are often mistaken regarding what women want, and that all women possess an unspoken connection—were born of an industry that kept women's faces healthy and beautiful. But they would also become ideas Evelyn would apply to the rest of a woman's body as well.

～

As the new American republic was being designed in 1776, Abigail Adams warned her husband, John (a future president), "If particular care and attention is not paid to the ladies, we are determined to foment a rebellion, and will not hold ourselves bound by any laws in which we have no voice or representation."[15]

And yet, since women were denied the ability to vote in governmental elections, representation was precisely what early American women lacked. By the mid-nineteenth century—just as Abigail had predicted—courageous women rebelled with a demand for suffrage.

Joining their sisters in Europe, the American suffragists' beliefs in social, economic, and political equality of the sexes earned them the label "feminists." Those who picketed, marched, and went on hunger strikes (along with occasional acts of vandalism and violence) also earned the label "radicals." And thus, even though there were less-demonstrative women who believed in equality, the term "feminism" took on a negative connotation. In truth, feminism has as many shades as the color blue. The women were persistent, and finally, in 1920, 144 years after Abigail Adams's warning, women won the right to vote.

Once women won the right to vote, the female mass mobilization, now known as the first wave of feminism, lost its unifying cause and fractured. Plus, with the stock market crash in 1929, the decade-long Great Depression that followed, and America's participation in World War II, most women did not have the time, the resources, or the energy to fight for anything more than survival.

When the war finally ended, the long-awaited prize of a return to "normal" family life emerged like a rainbow after a tempest. The men went back to work; the women went back to the home, cleaning, polishing, cooking, and reproducing. But a New York City woman wanted more. Betty Friedan had earned a bachelor's degree and was working as a journalist when she married in 1947. She returned to work after her first child was born, but when she became pregnant with the second, she was fired from her job because of the pregnancy, something employers could do to pregnant women until 1978.[16]

Friedan's active mind was restless while she was a full-time homemaker, and she wondered if other women felt the same. As a project for her fifteenth Smith College reunion, she sent out a questionnaire to sister alums, asking if they were using their education and if they were satisfied with their current lives. She was shocked by the passionate responses from many of the women, who were relieved to know they were not alone in asking themselves, "Is this all?"

When Friedan first published articles based on her findings, she called the women's dissatisfaction *it*, "the problem with no name." But by the time she published a book in February 1963, *it* had a name: the feminine mystique. Society, Friedan said, was pushing the notion that women were completely satisfied as wives, mothers, and homemakers—that was the feminine mystique. In reality, many were miserable, and then made to feel guilty for feeling so. The book was wildly popular among some, and savagely trashed by others.

The Feminine Mystique, combined with the report from Kennedy's Commission on the Status of Women that came out eight months later, became the tinder for the second wave of feminism. Even with the passage of the Civil Rights Act of 1964, which prohibited discrimination based on race, color, religion, sex, or national origin, very little changed in women's lives. Friedan and twenty-seven other sisters-in-arms founded the National Organization for Women (NOW). They proclaimed that "the time has come for a new movement toward true equality for all women in America."[17] But there was a problem.

In 1966, families had an average of 3.62 children.[18] Caring for them was a job most often performed by mothers. Juggling motherhood along with a job outside the home was difficult for women, and the childcare needed if a woman wanted to work outside the home could be costly. And while the traditional demands of equality—as in rights, pay, education, and more—were pressing, there could be no liberation without women being able to control their reproductive potential. In order for that to happen, women had to have a better understanding of their own bodies.

⟵

"I believe our country is in great trouble."[19] With that, Shirley Temple Black announced that she was running to represent California's Eleventh Congressional District. The seat, covering prosperous San Mateo County, a suburban spread south of San Francisco, had been vacated by the death of its former congressman.

Sixteen television cameras and twenty-two microphones captured Shirley's every word during the August 29, 1967, jam-packed press conference.

"The Great Society, a pretty bad movie in the first place, has become a great flop," Shirley continued.[20] And she wasted no words in criticizing the Great Society's architect, President Lyndon Johnson. Charging that he was playing politics with the Vietnam War, she pronounced that the end of the war had been delayed much too long. Shirley had a personal reason for wanting to hasten the war's end. Wedged in between her daughters on the speaker's platform—Susan, now nineteen and Lori, six years younger—was her son, Charles Black Jr. At fifteen and in military school, he was fast approaching draft age.

Running for political office was a new hat for Shirley, one of a number she had worn in her seventeen years of marriage to Charlie. Aside from being a wife and mother, she had thrown herself into charities as a tireless and dedicated volunteer. When her brother George was diagnosed with multiple sclerosis (MS) in 1951, she became the MS Society's director three years later, and the national chair of their 1960 Hope Chest fundraising campaign. With a foot still in acting, she narrated sixteen episodes of the NBC show *Shirley Temple's Storybook* from 1958 to 1961. But politics intrigued her.

During Richard Nixon's first run for the White House against John Kennedy, Shirley had guest-starred at rallies for him. On November 8, 1961, Nixon thanked her in a sentimental letter: "A year has gone by since our campaign of 1960 came to a close. I would not want this day to pass without taking the opportunity to tell you again how deeply grateful I am for all that you did for our cause."[21]

Shirley was frequently invited to speak for myriad organizations, and her topics evolved as her interests did. Having sampled the political waters in the course of some of her fundraising efforts, she realized she had important things to say about government spending and saving the environment. She was on her way home from sharing just such a message to a crowd of fifty thousand in a Houston arena when she realized how passionate she was about those issues. Equally important, it occurred to Shirley how much she enjoyed the prospect of sharing her passion in the hopes of persuading others. It was that speech that became the impetus for her entering the 1967 congressional race.

If Shirley thought, however, that she would receive the same welcome from the press in running for office as she had acting, she soon learned how wrong she was. Throughout her movie career, her mother and the studio had guarded her from harsh critiques. Now she was shocked by the journalists' viciousness. The opening sentence of nearly every article contained some version of "the onetime child movie star." This was followed by jabs at the titles of Shirley's movies. One article used the headline "Little Miss Candidate," a play on her 1934 movie *Little Miss Marker.*

The thirty-nine-year-old was defiant in addressing the reference to her first career, saying, "Little Shirley Temple isn't running. I have lived here for thirteen years and the people of this district know me as I am today."[22] But the demeaning career allusions continued, often accompanied by physical descriptions of her being "plump" and a "matron."

Shirley fought on. When election day rolled around on November 14, California had no congresswoman. That statistic remained unchanged when votes for Shirley came up short. The pioneering developer of the helicopter, Stanley Hiller, had served as her honorary campaign manager. After the votes were counted, he gave her two options: "You can either go home and close the door, or you can get on the road to help your party."

Shirley chose the latter, telling reporters after the loss, "I'm not going to give up. This is my first race and now I know how the game is played. I will be back."[23] She didn't have to wait long.

⟶

In the wee hours of Wednesday, November 6, 1968, Richard Milhous Nixon was finally proclaimed the thirty-seventh president of the United States. He received 55.9 percent of the Electoral College vote but won the popular vote by just 0.7 percent.[24] And when he took the oath of office on Monday, January 20, 1969, he inherited a nation in upheaval. The 1968 assassinations of Martin Luther King Jr. and Robert Kennedy were still fresh wounds to Americans' souls. Now, not far from the Capitol steps where Nixon was taking the oath of office, antiwar protests were heating up. Rocks and beer cans would later be hurled at the president's limousine during the inaugural parade. Like Kennedy and Johnson before him, Nixon became the new target for those opposing the Vietnam War.

During the campaign, Nixon had told journalist Theodore White, "I've always thought this country could run itself domestically without a president. You need a president for foreign policy."[25] But in 1969, domestic affairs couldn't be ignored. In addition to the antiwar movement, the civil rights movement, and its ensuing racial divisiveness, the women's movement had continued to grow.

At a press conference early in his administration the new president had been asked by journalist Vera Glaser, "Mr. President, since you've been inaugurated, you have made approximately two hundred presidential appointments, and only three of them have gone to women. Can we expect some more equitable recognition of women's abilities, or are we going to remain the lost sex?"[26]

Nixon was somewhat taken aback, and said, "We'll have to do something about that." Thus, the White House Task Force on Women's Rights and Responsibilities was created. It spent a year studying the situation, then made recommendations, which included that cabinet and agency heads should be directed to "issue firm instructions that qualified women receive equal consideration in hiring and promotion."[27]

The report's recommendations were not much different than those made by Kennedy's Commission on the Status of Women nearly a decade earlier. And they were certainly not what American women had hoped for. True, both presidents had essentially "remembered" the ladies, as Abigail Adams had requested. But neither remembered them with anything substantial in terms of equality with men. For Shirley, however, Nixon's need to uphold his task force's recommendations came at the perfect time.

She had made good on Stanley Hiller's suggestion after her election loss. "Shirley Says Declare War," shouted the *San Mateo Times* on February 20, 1968, quoting from a speech she had delivered.[28] It, and the speeches that followed, echoed those of then-candidate Nixon. Crisscrossing the country, she visited forty-six cities in twenty-two states, raising well over $1 million (over $9 million today) in support of the Republican candidate. Now that he was in the White House, she was hoping he'd remember the work she'd done on his behalf. It wasn't an outrageous expectation; diplomatic assignments, for example, often were handed out on the basis of what (and how much) individuals had done for presidents during their campaigns.

To start the conversation, and on behalf of the Multiple Sclerosis Society (whose national board she sat on), Shirley asked the president to be the honorary chair of the MS Society's 1969's fundraiser. He declined that, but did accept their Bronze Hope Chest award for that year. In advance of bestowing his award, Shirley sent a note asking for a few minutes with him after the May 20 Rose Garden ceremony. There were a number of positions in his administration that interested her, she told him, most specifically chief of protocol. No woman had ever held that position. Nixon, however, continued that tradition. She also wouldn't have minded being ambassador to the Netherlands, but that post went to a male investment banker.

An erroneous report circulated that she would be ambassador to the United Nations Educational, Scientific and Cultural Organization (UNESCO). However, on August 29, 1969, it was accurately reported that she had received a United Nations appointment. Again, the press wasted no time pulling out the daggers. Editorialist Robert Wiener wrote this assessment: "She is unschooled in geopolitics, innocent of the subtleties of diplomacy, provincial in viewpoint, untutored in history and graciously naive. She should fit right in."[29] Other journalists again began their stories with some version of "the curly-haired movie moppet" and "the onetime child movie star." Now, instead of "Little Miss Candidate," they wrote, she was "Little Miss Diplomat."

Letters of protest flooded into the White House: "She has no qualifications!" "You were wrong in appointing Shirley Temple Black." "Absolutely disgraceful." "Shirley Temple? You gotta be kidding."[30] The outcry wasn't helped by the fact that her actual position was never clearly explained. She was *a* representative to the U.N., not *the* representative. She was a part-timer, one of ten members of the United States delegation, as opposed to the career diplomats who hold their positions on a year-round basis. Her role was to attend the next General Session, beginning September 16, and represent the United States on the General Assembly's Social Committee. That committee handles "problems of the human environment," she explained to a reporter.[31] The same writer also thought it was necessary to include her swearing-in ceremony attire: "[She] wore an up-hairdo, a red suit, wore black pumps with rhinestones on the straps." Her male counterparts' outfits were never mentioned.

As annoying as the publicity might have been, her celebrity was actually a benefit in her new diplomatic career. She was known around the world. This drew people to her and allowed her to not only share her thoughts but learn from theirs as well. In addition, from the age of three, she had been a prodigy in terms of her confidence and ability to take command of any situation. Her co-stars had been awed by that quality. So employing it on the world stage came very naturally. As she would later say, "Shirley Temple opened doors for Shirley Temple Black."[32]

But if Shirley thought that, as a United Nations delegate, people would now see her only in her new role, she was mistaken. When she testified before a subcommittee of the House Committee on Foreign Affairs on February 26, 1970, New Jersey congressman Cornelius Gallagher giddily introduced her, saying, "I have long been a fan."[33]

Florida congressman J. Herbert Burke appeared to be an even bigger fan. "Mrs. Black," he said, "I just want you to know that I've seen *The Little Colonel* so many times that I expected you to walk in here wearing the uniform."[34]

And although the work she was about to do was of significant national importance, most articles covering it were buried in the women's sections of newspapers. But Shirley would not be deterred. She had made clear her interest in what would be the first-ever United Nations Conference on the Human Environment, to be held in Stockholm June 5–16, 1972. She was appointed to the preparatory committee, led by Christian A. Herter Jr. Herter was director of the State Department's Office of Environmental Affairs and would serve as vice chair of the U.S. delegation in Stockholm. She was the only woman, and Herter's insulting and dismissive attitude toward Shirley demonstrated his displeasure at not having a fully male committee.

When introductions were made around the table, Herter responded to each man, and then ignored Shirley. After those were out of the way, he turned to her and said with a patronizing smile, "And now, Madam Deputy, will you kindly take our requests for coffee? You can bring it from the machine down the hall."[35]

Shirley's appointment as part of the U.S. delegation at the Stockholm meeting would have been intimidating to anyone, even if they had spent time in the spotlight. Attendees included 1,200 delegates from 113 of the U.N.'s 132 member states. And as can be imagined, the conference was not all sunshine and lollipops. Nations that were adversaries, either under the radar or overtly, clashed verbally. It would have been natural for Shirley to be taken aback in those meetings. Yet her fellow delegates spoke afterward of her calm demeanor as she helped to smooth out bottlenecks in crafting the conference's concluding document, known as the Stockholm Declaration.

Speaking to the entire assemblage on the last day, Shirley appealed to world leaders beyond the four walls of the conference hall: "We aspire to live well in this earthly environment. But to do so, we must acknowledge our kinship as human beings, and the obligations of that kinship as the great law transcending nation, and ideology, and every other interest."[36] As it would into the future, the training from the first part of her life was guiding this chapter.

Shirley's success at the Stockholm conference earned her the next appointment: special assistant to the chairman of the Council on Environmental

Quality, part of the executive branch. Of the council's twenty-six members, she was again the only woman. She would be sworn in on September 1, 1972, and had taken a suite at the Jefferson Hotel in Washington, D.C. As she went through her morning regime, preparing for the Executive Office Building ceremony, Shirley performed a task she did religiously every day: a breast self-exam. Her gynecologist had recommended the then-new procedure soon after Susan was born in 1948. It had become so routine that Shirley was shocked when her fingers passed over the twelve o'clock position in her left breast and felt a lump.

In that moment, every woman reacts differently. In Shirley's case, there was really nothing she could do but finish dressing and go to the ceremony. But as soon as she returned to her hotel room, she called her doctor's office in California to make an appointment for immediately after she got home. "I wasn't really worried," she later said. "I don't know why."[37]

Shirley had known her doctor for a long time. He was a good friend, as well as a patient and "gifted man of medicine."[38] After assessing the lump and sending her for a mammogram (a still-new technology), he assured Shirley that there was a 60 percent chance it was nothing more than a cyst. The wise next step, he said, was to have it biopsied.

There were problems with that step. She was leaving for Moscow in a few weeks for her first assignment for the Council on Environmental Quality. There, she would meet with members of the council's USSR counterpart, the Soviet State Committee on Science and Technology. Then, the day after she returned stateside, she would be on her way to another environmental conference in Cincinnati. She wouldn't be back in California until early October. And the final hurdle was trying to mesh her schedule with that of the very busy Stanford University Medical Center doctor who would perform the biopsy, Frederic Shidler, who was also chief of surgery. The soonest date both could settle on was November 2, two months after she had first discovered the lump.

Besides understandable anxiety, it would have been perfectly natural if another thought crossed Shirley's mind. For five years, ever since she had run for a seat in Congress, Shirley had worked hard to show her male contemporaries that she was every bit as capable as they were in their work, *despite* being a woman. Now she was facing a very woman-centric condition in a part of the body never discussed in public. Regardless of whether Shirley's lump was cancer or not, women's vulnerability to breast disease might be regarded as yet another reason that women were too frail to participate in a man's world.

The lump didn't appear to grow larger, but it did begin to hurt. And once, while in Moscow, she was awakened by a tingling sensation in her breast. She recalled that her doctor had reassuringly told her of the 60 percent chance of the lump being benign. "Now," Shirley later wrote, "I began to feel as though I should be looking at the forty percent odds."[39]

And yet Shirley's optimism didn't wane. "It's strange how, at the last moment, what is mobilized is hope, not fear. One talks oneself into good news. It was probably nothing at all. They would take out a small benign lump and I would go home and then back to work in Washington."[40]

~

"What is to be done about cancer?"[41] In its May 1913 issue, *The Ladies' Home Journal* took the brave step of printing the word *cancer*, a word so frightening, journalists avoided writing it. The shocking article was written by Samuel Hopkins Adams, no stranger to controversial journalism. Eight years earlier he had penned "The Great American Fraud," an eleven-part series in *Collier's* magazine that exposed the many false claims made by patent medicine manufacturers.

One year after the 1912 sinking of the *Titanic*, tuberculosis and pneumonia were the top two causes of death in America. Cancer, Adams wrote, was third. Of every eight women who reached the age of thirty-five, one would die of the disease, along with one in eleven men. It was an irony, then, that while cancer strikes both sexes, this landmark article ran only in a women's magazine. It also nearly exclusively used the feminine pronouns "she" and "her" throughout.

In his query of nationally known cancer specialists (the term "oncology" wouldn't be in use for another half century), none could identify cancer's cause. Their advice—"sharp, positive and unanimous"—was to educate the people to save themselves. So Adams took up the charge.

"The fatalism which says, 'If it's cancer, I might as well give up,'" he wrote, "is foolish, cowardly and suicidal." He followed this with five warnings: no cancer is hopeless when discovered early; when discovered early, cancer is curable; medicines are worse than useless (referring to the "snake oil" products widely advertised); delay is more than dangerous, it is deadly; and the only cure is the knife. Chemotherapy and radiation treatments were decades off. Surgery was the sole option for patients, and it, too, was often feared by the general public. The idea of entering the human body via an incision, coupled with the dread of pain and the real possibility of infection, was nearly as terrifying as cancer itself.

Adams also pointed to European doctors' then-unparalleled success in treating cancer. For all of America's industrial might in the early days of the twentieth century, the country lagged sorrowfully in medical advances. The United States was so far behind, in fact, that most young American doctors took their postgraduate training in Berlin, Munich, and other prominent European cities. "The German physician has benefited by the general enlightenment," Adams stated, "and is better skilled in recognizing the early stages of the malady."

In closing his two-page story, he included a stern warning from Dr. Charles H. Mayo, whom he called one of the greatest surgeons in America: "The risk is not in surgery, but in *delayed* surgery."

Chapter 4

An Amputation

"Have you ever been paid less than a man?" "Have you ever resented . . . that almost all the important political decisions are made by a man?" "Have you ever had to give up a cherished hope or ambition because it was 'unfeminine?'"[1]

The one-page typewritten sheet listed these and seven other questions referring to the myriad ways in which women were discriminated against in 1970. Next to each was the opportunity to circle yes or no.

The page continued. "You do not have to be a militant feminist or 'women's liberationist' or a man-hater or a bra burner. If you are a woman who has ever felt that she is not quite a first class citizen because she is female, you must demonstrate that fact on August 26."

That date was significant. Exactly fifty years before, the Nineteenth Amendment had given women the right to vote, but very little had changed in the ensuing years. Therefore, any woman who was able to answer yes to even one of the questions was urged to join the Women's Strike for Equality on that day, staying home from her job and not undertaking "menial household tasks."

The last line on the page was printed in capital letters: "IF YOU DO NOTHING, YOU ARE SAYING THAT YOU ARE TOTALLY SATISFIED WITH YOUR INFERIOR STATUS."

The scene that ultimately occurred on August 26, 1970, was historic, and beyond what organizers Betty Friedan and the other members of NOW could have imagined. More than twenty thousand women marched down New York

City's Fifth Avenue, demanding their rights at home, in the classroom, and at the office. Marches also took place in Boston, Chicago, Indianapolis, and forty other American cities, as well as in France and the Netherlands. The ages, ethnicities, and social classes of the marchers spanned the gamut; it wasn't just a radical few who were unhappy. As had been necessary for the women of the first wave of feminism, a new unifying cause had been found by their daughters and granddaughters. And before long, the bedrock of the second wave of feminism was established: consciousness-raising groups.

The concept was simple. Women came together with the united purpose of enhancing their consciousness about their feminine identity. They started talking, sharing stories, discussing challenges. This clearly feminine act—coming together to share their feelings—was something that threatened men often sought to suppress.

Inevitably, the groups' discussions landed on their most uniting element of all, their femaleness. There were those who had no idea how their reproductive systems worked. And there were those who knew but had never seen the living parts, either theirs or anyone else's. But this gynecological ignorance was about to end.

Armed with flashlights, mirrors, and speculums, consciousness-raising group leaders showed the rest of the attendees how to examine their own bodies. What they saw was not something dark, foul, and mysterious, as had been suggested of female genitalia for centuries. Rather, these women saw what was responsible for the continuation of the species. And it was beautiful. As Ellen Frankfort wrote in her 1972 book, *Vaginal Politics,* "It was like having a blind person see for the first time."[2]

Paving the road for "the blind" had begun at tiny Emmanuel College in Boston. Over the weekend of May 10–11, 1969 (just five months after Nixon's first electoral win), the college hosted the New England Regional Female Liberation Conference. A variety of workshops were planned, including on music, writing, interracial marriages, and more, with self-defense demonstrations also provided each day.

On Sunday the eleventh, at 10:00 a.m., a two-hour workshop was on the agenda, entitled "Women and Their Bodies."[3] Only eight white middle-class women came (although an unexpected total of five hundred women attended the conference as a whole). The workshop leader had just had a baby two weeks earlier, so their discussions naturally covered childbirth, sexuality, relationships, birth control, and abortions. They also discussed unpleasant encounters with doctors. Those encounters were not, they discovered, random occurrences, or the result of anything the women themselves had done. Rather, it appeared that this was just one more problem women faced. The small group vowed to ignite change, and the movement was born.

Calling themselves "the doctor's group," their first step was to identify physicians willing to be open with them. When those brave doctors began to educate them on what they didn't know about the female anatomy, they realized that the next step had to be spending the summer researching the areas they had discussed in that earlier workshop. Reuniting a few months later, they shared their findings, wrote up reports to assemble into a book, and rebranded themselves as the Boston Women's Health Book Collective. When college resumed in the fall of 1969, the collective organized a meeting in a student lounge at the Massachusetts Institute of Technology. Mimeographed copies of their "book" were distributed to the attendees.

From that groundbreaking workshop, many of the participants volunteered to take the information to other women. The process began replicating itself across the country, just as the collective had hoped, but faster than they ever imagined. It was time to create a proper book. In December 1970, they published five thousand copies of *Women and Their Bodies*. Printed on newsprint and stapled together, fifteen thousand more copies of the 193-page book were in print in April 1971. By the time they retitled the book as *Our Bodies, Ourselves* in 1973, 350,000 copies were in circulation. (Revised, updated, and reprinted until 2011, over four million copies of *Our Bodies, Ourselves* have been sold.)

And women who had previously been passive recipients of healthcare began to ask themselves, "if such knowledge and truth had previously been unavailable to them, what else were the medical men—94% of gynecologists were male in the 1970s—hiding?"[4] At that moment a lightbulb turned on for many. Not only had women been assigned to "proper" gender roles in all other aspects of their daily lives, but they were expected to maintain their proper place in the physician-patient relationship as well.

In gynecological exams across the country, women disrobed, covered themselves with a sheet, and drew up their knees to place their feet in stirrups. Not only did the doctor often not look at the woman attached to the nether parts he was examining, but the woman couldn't see what the doctor was doing. That sheet was the symbol of the veil of secrecy. A female patient had the duty to do what she was told. The *doctor* had attended medical school. The *doctor* had knowledge. The *doctor* wasn't to be questioned. Even television promulgated the myth of the physician as God. In *Dr. Kildare* (debuting in 1961), *Marcus Welby, M.D.* (1969), *Emergency* (1972), and other shows, the physicians saved the day, the nurses cleaned up, and the patients either smiled mutely or died.

Similar scenes also played out when a woman presented with a suspicious lump in her breast. Nearly always being "calmed" with the words "It's probably nothing," she was told to make an appointment with a surgeon and plan for an overnight hospital stay. On the appointed day, and terrified at the notion that she might have cancer, the woman gladly signed the documents put before her when she arrived, as if her signature alone might remove the potential of cancer. Rather, it removed so much more.

The one thing Shirley knew for certain was that she would not be one of the thousands of women who, lying inert on an operating table for a biopsy, allowed a team of strangers to make a decision that would affect the rest of her life. "For those who wanted it that way, okay," she later wrote. "For those who had fate snatched from their own hands against their will, my great sympathy."[5]

When Wednesday, November 1, rolled around, Shirley packed an overnight bag and drove alone to the Stanford University Hospital, fifteen minutes away from her home in Woodside, California. Biopsies were a surgical event in that era, requiring patients to spend the night before and, if cancer was found, afterward. The next morning, before she was wheeled into the operating room, Shirley signed an agreement for an excisional biopsy only. She understood fully that a doctor's mission was to save lives. But she was insistent that while the doctor could make the *in*cision, she would make the final *de*cision about her own breast. This was an unheard-of request in 1972. And had she not been who she was, complete with a diplomat's skill at politely making herself heard, she might not have gotten away with it.

A few hours later, as Shirley climbed through an anesthesia-induced haze, Charlie's face came into view, just as it had after her rushed appendectomy twelve years earlier.

"Darling," he said, "they got the tumor out and it was very small. Everything is just fine except for a tiny piece at one end of it that's malignant."[6] His face faded as she dozed off.

When she awoke again, a young doctor—probably a resident, as Stanford is a teaching hospital—was standing at the end of the bed, scanning a chart. When he saw she was awake, he said, "Mrs. Black, the tumor is malignant and we have to remove the breast."[7]

"I don't think so," Shirley replied groggily. "You just talk to my surgeon and he will tell you that everything is fine."

"I have talked to your surgeon," the doctor replied.

Again Shirley slipped into sleep. When she awoke a third time, her mind was sharper and the reality of the situation hit her full-on. She cried, and when her daughters arrived, they all cried together.

Dr. Shidler had told Charlie that Shirley's two-centimeter tumor (a little under an inch) was about six weeks old. That was a curious statement, since even today it is difficult to ascertain when a tumor first appeared. The statement is even more curious given that it was actually eight weeks since she had found the lump. Nevertheless, that comment hit Shirley hard. Perhaps, she thought, if she had seen to it earlier, she would have been spared what would come next.

Still, Shidler was reasonably sure that the cancer had not spread to her axillary (underarm) lymph nodes. This was good news. He and his team recommended a modified radical mastectomy to be performed the next day. They would remove Shirley's breast, along with all the lymph nodes, just to be safe. They would not, however, take muscle or bone, although that was part of the standard procedure at the time.

For better or worse, the lymphatic system serves as a highway for the body. Its network of nodes (clumped like tiny bunches of grapes) and vessels carries off waste products, bacteria, and cellular debris. The system is also one of the avenues that opportunistic cancer cells use on their march to other body parts. Removal of those nodes, however, is not without adverse effects, as fluids back up; when lymph nodes near a breast are removed, that can result in swelling of the arm on the affected side.

Breast cancer information available to the general public (even someone with Shirley's connections) was sparse. In advance of her biopsy, Shirley had read the only book she could find, written by a surgeon named George Crile Jr. She had absorbed everything in it and articles she found, and this much she knew: removing all of her lymph nodes without the certainty of cancer didn't make sense. The diplomat again politely but insistently voiced her resolute position. Since her doctors didn't believe the cancer was in her nodes, a compromise was in order. The surgical team would perform a simple mastectomy the next day, removing only her breast. If they saw something that would cause them to believe the cancer had spread beyond her breast, then, and *only* then, did she consent to the removal of her lymph nodes.

⸺

The Greek physician Hippocrates was at the ground floor of medicine's understanding of cancer, as he had been with hysteria. In fact, if it were not for him, cancer might have had any number of other names. In examining tumors removed from cadavers, Hippocrates couldn't help but compare their irregular shapes to crabs, with tentacles reaching out in all directions. Crab is *karkinos* in Greek, and the word eventually evolved into the English *carcinoma*.

Five hundred years later, around A.D. 175, another Greek physician, Galen, added his observation. He described the tumors he took from cadavers as *oncos*, or swollen. That term would also find its way into the medical vocabulary to describe a cancer specialist: an oncologist. Believing that incurable cancer was caused by thick black bile, while a curable version of the disease came from thin yellow bile, Galen devised treatments to eliminate both types. He employed a cornucopia of ingredients to rub on visible tumors, or to ingest if the tumor couldn't be seen, accompanying his pharmaceutical treatments with bloodletting and inducing vomiting and diarrhea. All were popular procedures of his time, if only randomly successful.

Early beliefs about the causes of breast cancer seem equally far-fetched today. Perhaps patients had ingested curdled milk or suffered from depression. Their sexual activity might have created a lymphatic blockage, and their tumors were actually pus-filled inflammations that mingled with blood. Some doctors claimed a sedentary lifestyle caused breast cancer, while others pointed to being childless as the problem, thus giving way to the moniker "nun's disease." (The latter was not that far off, in that modern medicine lists never having borne a child as a potential risk factor.)

But regardless of cause, it eventually became obvious that the sole remedy to save a woman's life was the knife. Mastectomies (the word again derived from the Greek *mastos*, referring to a woman's breast, and the Latin *ectomia*, meaning "excision") had become favored as breast cancer treatment in the early 1600s among German surgeons. The French followed suit a century later. The custom was to do the surgery *en bloc*, removing the breast as a whole entity, to ensure no particle of tumor could escape and settle elsewhere.

Over time, surgeons devised a variety of tools to lift the breast off the chest wall before cutting it off. Forceps were used to pinch and constrict the breast. Alternatively, large fishhooks were attached to ropes and inserted on either side of the breast. Pulling the ropes raised the breast, allowing a surgeon to cut and cauterize with hot irons as he went. All of these procedures were done without anesthesia.

In the nineteenth century, four important pioneers changed breast cancer surgery forever. British doctor Joseph Lister discovered that microbes caused infection. He began cleansing his hands, instruments, and the patients' bodies with carbolic acid before surgery. (When his discovery was later made available for sale by Dr. Joseph Lawrence, he called it Listerine in homage to Lister.) Meanwhile, American dentist William Morton was called into an operation to remove a facial tumor. He successfully used the ether he had previously employed during dental procedures, illustrating that doctors would no longer have to stare into the eyes of their terrified, moaning, conscious patients.

At the same time in Prussia, Rudolf Virchow, known as the "father of modern pathology," compared normal and abnormal tissues. He concluded that cancer was the result of a cellular disorder, paving the way for surgeons to be able to discern benign tumors from malignant ones.

The fourth pioneer's discovery also changed surgical procedures and lives, but not without consequences. American doctor William Stewart Halsted was born in 1852. He was a brilliant student and a brilliant surgeon. Although addicted to cocaine, he was a high-functioning addict.[8] The discoveries of the first three pioneers gave Halsted the opportunity to do precision surgery without worry for the woman's pain, and the confidence that he was taking away diseased tissue without concern that infection would ultimately kill the patient. But women were still dying. Cancer cells were apparently remaining after their mastectomies.

Halsted had read papers written by a British contemporary, Charles Moore, whose experience taught him that a return of breast cancer almost always occurred around the edges of the original surgery. Not taking enough tissue, Moore said, was a "mistaken kindness."[9] Halsted took this to heart, resolving to get to the root of the cancer with a technique called radical mastectomy (*radical* is Latin for "root"). In 1894, he performed the first. His *en bloc* procedure required removal not only of the breast but also of all the axillary lymph nodes, the pectoralis minor muscle, and the pectoralis major (the muscle responsible for shoulder and hand movement), along with the overlying skin.

It was true, Halsted acknowledged, that his radical mastectomies created unavoidable physical challenges afterward. But he had achieved a momentous goal. His patients' five-year survival rate was 40 percent, twice that of patients who hadn't undergone his radical mastectomies.[10] And if cancer did return, so would Halsted's knife, carving into patients' rib cages and collarbones.

⚯

Someone was calling Shirley's name. She was pulled from sleep to see it was a nurse. "Did you do it?" Shirley asked. "Yes," the nurse said, "the breast has been removed."[11] As before, Shirley again drifted in and out of sleep. During one of her wakeful moments, she allowed her right hand to touch the void on the left side of her chest. *This is an amputation,* she thought.

By Sunday, November 5, the patient was feeling astonishingly more chipper. When her family arrived, she told them that she'd been pondering how she could turn her experience into something helpful for her "sisters," as she called them. While a relatively private person, Shirley knew her celebrity would offer the opportunity to reach hundreds of thousands of women. She might be able to help those who were in the same situation as she was. And, just as important, she might help those diagnosed with breast cancer down the road.

In movies, Shirley had often played characters who faced their challenges with optimism and a can-do spirit. As America had grappled with the harsh realities of the Great Depression, Shirley reminded audiences that despite dark times, there was room for joy and laughter. Even President Franklin Roosevelt saw that. "It is a splendid thing," he said, "that for just 15 cents, an American can go to a movie and look at the smiling face of a baby and forget his troubles!"[12]

As a young woman, Shirley had visited hospitals filled with recovering soldiers, sailors, and pilots who had been injured in World War II and joined her fellow actors entertaining at USO shows. And when her brother George was diagnosed with multiple sclerosis, she jumped into fundraising and awareness campaigns. The world had needed Shirley Temple when she was a movie screen regular. Now, she reasoned, breast cancer survivors needed her, too.

Shirley's first call was to her son, Charlie junior, who was on a fishing boat off Panama, to let him know of her plan. Next she called Dave Shutz, a family friend and editor of their local newspaper. He was shocked to hear about her cancer, and even more so when he came to see her in the hospital.[13] She presented him with her statement, breaking every rule of the "never" world in which they lived: *Never* mention the word cancer aloud. *Never* speak about your own breasts, especially in public. (You could, however, show off your breasts, with or without clothing.) And, as a celebrity, *never* discuss medical problems with reporters. To the contrary, hide them.

⁓

Since the 1940s, Mary Lasker had become a familiar face in the halls of congressional office buildings, as well as in the hearing rooms where medical research funds were doled out. She and her husband, Albert Lasker, the millionaire father of modern advertising (he would be a billionaire by today's standards), reimagined the American Society for the Control of Cancer. The society was surviving on a minuscule annual budget of $50,000 in 1943. The Laskers changed its name to the American Cancer Society, increased its fundraising to produce millions annually, and debuted its support of medical research.

When her husband died of cancer in 1952, Mary's anti-cancer mission became a crusade. She counted senators, congressmen, and presidents from both sides of the aisle among her friends, including all of the Kennedys. However, Richard Nixon wasn't one of them; she was anything but a fan of his and not happy about his 1968 election.

In March 1971, Mary contacted Senator Ted Kennedy to suggest that he introduce a bill to accelerate cancer research. It would remove the bureaucratic hurdles that the National Cancer Institute had to navigate. It would fast-track research from laboratory benches to patients in hospital beds. It would create the National Cancer Advisory Board (NCAB), a group of medical professionals *and* laypeople who would oversee the NCI's progress, reporting directly to the president. And it would infuse an unheard-of amount of money to support that research: more than $1 billion ($7.7 billion today). These were radical but crucial demands.

When President Nixon realized the accolades Kennedy would receive if the bill succeeded, he jumped at the chance to be the cancer-slayer in chief. The political wrangling that occurred between the two men and their respective parties continued for nine months. In the end, on December 23, 1971, the president gleefully signed the National Cancer Act, calling it his "Christmas gift to the nation."[14] For her part, Mary said Nixon might turn out "to be the most sympathetic president we've ever had."[15] Politics aside, the National Cancer Act changed the future for every cancer patient around the world.

It was too soon for Shirley Temple's mastectomy procedure to have been affected by Nixon's signature 315 days earlier. But she would effect a great change for breast cancer survivors nonetheless. In 1972, most cancer patients weren't keen to share information about their diagnoses beyond their immediate families. And sometimes even families were left in the dark. Conversely, because cancer was so often fatal, patients weren't always told they had it.

Cancer's unkind stigmas, such as the notion that the disease resulted from uncleanliness or bad lifestyle choices, were damaging enough. But worst of all was the persistent though erroneous belief that cancer was contagious. Prior to the twentieth century, nearly all of the world's most deadly illnesses fell into that category. Bubonic plague, smallpox, cholera, tuberculosis, and many others took children and adults with abandon. Whether spread by air, water, or bodily fluids, plagues and epidemics taught humans a valuable lesson: stay away from someone who is sick.

Now Shirley, one of the world's best-known women, was inviting people into her private life to discuss a very private part of her body. She was also inviting the press into her hospital room, potentially swimming with "cancer germs." And yet on Monday, November 6, the press came. She was the first, *ever,* to go public with her breast cancer.

In front of lights, cameras, and reporters busily scribbling notes, Shirley began her groundbreaking account of how she had found her own cancer. She looked beautiful, her makeup done to perfection, her hair styled with a gardenia pinned at her right ear. She wore a slightly off-the-shoulder nightgown, with the bedsheet demurely pulled up, covering her chest.[16]

"It is my fervent hope," Shirley said as she finished her three-minute statement, "that women will not be afraid to go to their doctors when they have unusual symptoms."

The scrum of reporters then began asking questions. How did she feel? How had she found the lump? Did she regularly do breast self-exams? The topic of this press conference was a world away from the one that congressional candidate Shirley Temple Black had done five years earlier, but this time around she answered each question with the same calm conviction in her beliefs and decisions as she had then.

Because of the time difference, only the California press was able to get this earth-shattering news into their Monday evening papers. But by the next morning, the whole country knew what Shirley had been through. That day, Tuesday, November 7, happened to also be election day. President Nixon was on the ballot for his second term. Feeling positive about the results (he ultimately would win in a landslide), while he waited for the final vote count he sent Shirley one of the first telegrams she received after the press conference.

"Pat and I were distressed to learn of your surgery." (Even the president couldn't bring himself to say the word *cancer*.) "And we just want you to know that you are in our thoughts and prayers at this time. We hope you are resting comfortably, and we send you our very best wishes for a full and prompt recovery. With our warmest regards, Richard Nixon."[17]

Then came the deluge. The Stanford University Medical Center switchboard fielded thousands of phone calls. Flower arrangements overtook Shirley's room, so she began distributing them to other patients. Sacks of letters and telegrams flooded in, numbering over fifty thousand by the time she went home.[18] The messages came from all over the world, Shirley noted, "including the Congo." They were moving and unexpected.

"Your decision to let the public know of your mastectomy is one of the rare instances of a public personality making a completely unselfish decision."

"We—you and I, and all others like us—are fortunate to have been endowed with a wonderful gift . . . a second chance to fully enjoy what we came so close to losing."

"I no longer feel so lonely in my own misery because I know I share my misfortune with a famous and beautiful lady."

One wire particularly filled her with love: "I offer you my prayer of thanks to the Almighty God for having saved your life also. . . . Way back in 1944, I had the unforgettable privilege of meeting you briefly at Letterman General Hospital in San Francisco. I was a disabled veteran just returning from the front."[19]

In a second trailblazing move, Shirley began writing a four-page magazine article as soon as she got home from the hospital, on November 12. It appeared three months later in the February 1973 issue of *McCall's,* one of the most widely read women's magazines in the country. The final lines left no one wondering about what she hoped for the readers: "Leave the questions of beauty and vanity aside. In a well-balanced existence, these are unworthy virtues. Consider instead, as I do, the more fundamental virtues of enthusiasm, intellectual vigor and the unquenchable desire to serve others until the final bell rings. With or without a breast, I plan to keep doing precisely what I have been doing. Only better."[20]

Shirley's goal for the press conference and magazine article had been to motivate the more than seventy thousand women who would be diagnosed with breast cancer in 1973. More than one-third of them might have died because, as she wrote, after finding something unusual in their breast, "they failed to face up *in time* to the hard but manageable reality." A few weeks after her press conference and the flurry of newspaper reports it unleashed, Shirley received proof that her goal had been achieved at least once. A woman wrote a note saying that initially she had been shocked that any woman would discuss such a "personal" subject as the removal of a breast. The announcement had caused her to move her hand to her own breast, where she discovered a lump. She was now writing from a hospital in Oakland, California, awaiting her biopsy the next day. The letter ended with heartfelt gratitude. Shirley had potentially saved her life.[21]

But Shirley's crusade was just getting started. Television was her next target. She had been on Dinah Shore's show twice in 1972. (Dinah was a singer and actress before launching her daytime program. She would die of ovarian cancer twenty-two years later.) Shirley's first appearance was on September 27; at that time, only she and Charlie knew about the lump in her breast. The episode's description was an odd stew: "Shirley Temple Black prepares scallops with wine sauce, and discusses pollution and her trip to Russia."[22]

The episode of Shirley's second interview, on October 31 (also before anyone else knew about her lump), had an equally incongruous description. "Shirley Temple Black talks about her recent trip to the Soviet Union. She and Dinah sample Russian foods, and Dinah sings 'Moscow Nights.'" But when she appeared on January 30, 1973, the description had far more significance. "Shirley Temple Black talks about her recent surgery for breast cancer, and answers questions from the audience on cancer prevention and detection."[23]

Shirley's next small-screen visit was to *The Mike Douglas Show,* appearing on May 25, 1973. The format of the twelve-year-old daytime program generally featured a weekly co-host—forty-six-year-old Tony Bennett was serving in the capacity that week—airing on stations around the country. Joining Shirley was a lanky and quiet Muhammad Ali (then thirty-one), who asked for her autograph during a commercial break. Also on the set was twenty-two-year-old Lorna Luft, Liza Minelli's half-sister, who made mention that Shirley had been considered for the part that her mother, the late Judy Garland, had been awarded in *The Wizard of Oz.*

After some small talk, Douglas asked Shirley if they could talk about her cancer. As candid as she had been in her press conference, magazine article, and previous TV appearances, she explained finding the lump, the biopsy, and the mastectomy.

"I'm confused," Douglas said. "Before the biopsy, don't you sign a paper of some kind?"[24]

"Well, that's where we sort of parted company, the hospital and me," Shirley replied. "I said I would sign a paper for the biopsy. But I didn't want them to go farther until I knew the results of that biopsy. After all, it's my body, I felt I should be part of the decision." Like the shot at Fort Sumter, that was a statement heard around the world.

It was another revolutionary first for Shirley. No woman had ever suggested or discussed—especially in such a public way—that a biopsy and a mastectomy be separate procedures. Just as the "doctor's group" (that small group of women in Boston) had discovered in 1969, women were still being expected to sign agreements for the amputation of their breasts; no further discussion was expected, much less any challenge.

Douglas was mesmerized by Shirley's calm and candor. "I sit here and listen to this courageous woman who's talking about this, with a smile on her face. And I'm thinking about how I would react to something like that. Because I went through this with my brother. It's something I don't know if I could cope with myself." Douglas's brother, Bob, had died of cancer four years earlier.

Shirley, however, had no doubt about Douglas's courage. "Of course you could!" she insisted.

He wasn't convinced. "But when the moment comes—" he began, and then abruptly changed the subject, asking about the content of the letters Shirley had received after making her announcement.

Shirley obliged, recounting the story of a British woman who, with her husband, had recently returned to their parked car to find it surrounded by police. Apparently a thief had meant to rob the car, but when he found a prosthetic breast and a hairpiece, he called the police to come look for the rest of the body that he was certain had been dismembered.

After the laughter died down, Shirley offered a sober observation. "The operation is ugly and maiming. I don't mean to make light of it. It wasn't having cancer that bothered me. It was losing an old friend."

In that moment F. Scott Fitzgerald's quote "There are no second acts in life" was disproven. While journalists insisted that Shirley's diplomatic career was her "second act," clearly her role as a beacon for her "sisters" was her *real* second act. It was the one that mattered most, and it signaled the beginning of the breast cancer movement.

Another pioneering breast cancer warrior would later also make a stop on Douglas's show. The celebrated soul singer Minnie Riperton had been diagnosed in 1976, undergoing a mastectomy (no doubt radical), despite knowing that her cancer had already spread. She continued touring and performing, and became a national spokeswoman for the American Cancer Society. On June 15, 1979, Minnie made her last televised appearance with Douglas, performing and being interviewed. She died less than a month later, at the age of thirty-one.[25]

~

There had been a threat of rain on Sunday, June 3, 1972. But the cloudy skies never touched Rose Kushner's demeanor. After twenty-six years of fits and starts, she had finally done it: she was about to graduate from college. Rose wasn't the typical University of Maryland graduate sitting in the Cole Student Activities Building that morning.[26] In addition to the length of time it had taken her to get there, and the fact that her husband and three children were cheering her on (Gantt was now twenty, Todd was sixteen, and Lesley was fourteen), she was graduating summa cum laude. Along with that high honor, she had also won the Sigma Delta Chi regional award, bestowed for excellence by the Society of Professional Journalists.

The award was most deserving, given the prolific amount of writing Rose had done over the past decade. Her brother Ike was well settled in his career at the *Baltimore Sun*. His way of telling a story made it look easy, making him the perfect mentor. Rose clearly shared his skills, along with honing a number of her own.

Rose's journalistic interests varied and evolved over time. Her first articles appeared in Jewish newspapers and magazines. "I would be delighted to have a witty or humorous article for the Passover issue," the editor of the *American Jewish Times-Outlook* said in answer to her query letter.[27] "Most of this magazine will be information and articles which will be somewhat dry—something light would break the monotony of the reading." That was all Rose needed to hear. She turned on her well-developed sense of humor, delighting not only the editor but the readers as well.

A subject that increasingly drew her in, however, was the same one that dominated every newspaper in the country: the Vietnam War. In 1961, President Kennedy had sent five hundred Special Forces troops, along with a cadre of military advisors, to the country. But it was President Johnson's multiplication of that number in 1965 (despite his campaign promises to the contrary) that made Americans sit up and take notice.

Rose had been intrigued in June 1967 by the way Israel had managed to win, in her view, "the hearts and minds" of its Arab adversaries, deescalating hostilities in what came to be known as the Six-Day War. The psychological warfare they used drew on principles similar to what she had learned in Dr. Gantt's lab: if desired behavior is rewarded, it's likely to be repeated. Consequently, Rose felt that America's increasing failure to win and exit the war in Vietnam was neither military nor political but psychological.[28]

Retired Air Force Major General Edward Lansdale agreed. The Central Intelligence Agency had made him the senior liaison officer at the American Embassy in Saigon. His work had been described as "mythical" and "legendary." To Rose and her family, he was simply their friend Ed, whom they had met a number of years earlier. She was such a fan of his, in fact, she began writing *Peace Hawks*, a book detailing his work. And she decided a research trip to Vietnam was essential to gain credibility for the book.[29]

"I'm just a Montgomery County housewife," she described herself when she arrived in Saigon in October 1967. But it didn't take long for Rose's inquisitiveness to half-amuse, half-intimidate the U.S. officials there. Upon her arrival, she had asked the spokesman then in charge of psychological warfare, "How many psychologists are working for you?" Her blunt question shocked him into honesty, and he replied, "None." That, she surmised, was problem number one for the psychological warfare program.[30]

Execution of that program was the other problem, causing her to sputter later in a newspaper article, "We're rewarding people who don't deserve rewards and punishing those who don't deserve to be punished."[31] She perceived it as the opposite of Pavlov's thesis that she had watched Dr. Gantt employ in his lab. America's response to the growing war was "cock-eyed," she said. Rose was convinced that the tide would turn if America offered the Vietnamese people everything the communists were offering them, plus freedom.

The Vietnamese, however, only saw the Americans defoliating their farmlands and relocating them to refugee camps, and they worried about ultimate annihilation as the Americans' possible end game. This angered Rose. Innocent people should not be pushed around by bullies. Given that her family had once escaped persecution by the totalitarian Russian regime, she knew all about bullies, so in a sense what was happening in Vietnam was personal to her.

One of the people Rose befriended in Vietnam was Lt. General Nguyen Chanh Thi, who, among other things, had been outspoken about his government's corruption. While Thi was on what was meant to be a short trip to Washington, D.C., the South Vietnamese decided not to allow Thi to return home. Viewing him as another poor soul being bullied, Rose tried to help him through the governmental contacts she had established. While waiting for responses, she kept his spirits up with cocktail parties, attended by other expats around D.C. She'd put on full Jewish deli spreads for them, washed down with a river of American cocktails.

Rose's mind was a constant swirl of ideas for her writing, which set her fingers flying across the typewriter keys to put those ideas on paper. She asked questions and was fearless in seeking out people who knew things that she wanted to know, including Israeli military leader and politician Moshe Dayan, Secretary of State Henry Kissinger, and CIA chief William Colby.

Colby, as it happened, moored his thirty-seven-foot sailboat, *Eagle Wing II*, in an Annapolis marina slip next to the Kushners' *Wind Song*. The Kushners rarely used the sails, however. Harvey—as the captain—was good at giving sailing orders. Rose—as the mate—wasn't good at taking them. To avoid the ensuing arguments, the family compromised by motoring everywhere they went, or just hung out on the boat in its slip, partying with their boating neighbors.[32]

As the months (and then years) passed, while she waited for *Peace Hawks* to be picked up by a publisher, Rose's Vietnam experiences became seeds for a stage play called *Wind Shadows* and a musical comedy called *Magyari!* Neither the book nor the scripts saw the light of day, but Rose was undeterred. She kept plugging away with enthusiasm, drawing on her own past experiences. "Writers write," she said. "Everything is a story."[33]

Chapter 5

⟡

A Streak of Stubbornness
and a Loud Voice

The beauty industry that the Lauders worked in every day was anything but beautiful. Rival brands, including Dorothy Gray, Helena Rubenstein, Revlon, and Elizabeth Arden, launched attacks on every side. The brands vied for counter space and position in the cosmetics department (nearest to the front door was premium). Research and development of new products were guarded like state secrets. And Evelyn loved it all, relishing her position at the creational ground floor of advanced skin care products and the ever-changing Estée Lauder makeup line.

Thirty years before, Helena Rubinstein had proclaimed cosmetics as vital in a woman's life. During World War II, however, her products had been criticized as unnecessary during such a period of hardship. Rubinstein argued to the contrary—that in "times of trouble and depression, women needed the added lift of makeup." She claimed that President Franklin Roosevelt had agreed, telling her, "Your war effort . . . is to help keep up the morale of our women. And you are doing it splendidly."[1]

Evelyn held the same belief as her rival, saying that while women enjoyed being complimented by men and other women who saw the results of their skin care and makeup regimen, "first and foremost you do it for your own confidence level."[2]

As invigorated as the corporate world made her feel, Evelyn was even more thrilled with motherhood. Early on, she taught William and Gary to mine for the real gold in life: "Money comes and money goes. But what you do have with you forever is your character and your education."[3] Of course, not every child in New York City had a positive and supportive mother. Neither did they have exciting and safe places to be just who they were: kids.

Leonard was picking the boys up at a Central Park playground one day when he realized that nothing had changed there since he was a child decades earlier. Patches of asphalt were surrounded by chain-link fence. The seesaws and swings were dangerous, when they functioned at all. There was no grass and no trees, but there were plenty of signs with the word *no*, most of which referred to the very things kids like to do. Furthermore, as New York became less and less child-friendly, parents began fleeing with their families to the suburbs.[4]

What was needed was a playground, Leonard thought, something created at a reasonable price that would not only serve the children but also keep the city vibrant. It would be a win-win for everyone. He talked to Evelyn, who was completely on board. They tapped architect Richard Dattner, the designer of their company's Long Island factory. Brainstorming with him, they came up with a rough design that the Lauders then took to the city parks commissioner, who loved it. Better still, no city money would be used. Estée and Joe had just launched a foundation, and the Lauders promised that they would fund not just one park but three.

The city, the foundation, the architect, and a mothers' committee made up of women from the neighborhoods surrounding the park went to work. When Adventure Playground opened in May 1967, the $85,000 park got rave reviews from parents, as well as from the toughest critics of all, the kids themselves. City children didn't have a creek to wade in like their country counterparts. But there was an artificial one at the park, along with a sprinkler pad so they could play in the "rain."[5] A giant-step pyramid allowed them to climb, and tunnels sent them exploring. The enormous sandbox was perfect for digging and castle construction. The kids became a blur of activity, with the adults having just as much fun watching them. And it was all repeated in two more parks, as promised.

Estée was thrilled with the public's reaction. "If a child is happy, it influences his life as an adult," she told a reporter philosophically. More than that, it was the first time a beauty company gave back to a city that had given them so much. Plus there was an added bonus: it was good for business. As another reporter observed, "The playground makes a woman feel justified paying $5 for a lipstick." (That would be $47 today.)[6]

Evelyn viewed the playground's success philosophically, too. As part of a now $15 million company, she had developed an ever-increasing need to give back to the country where she felt her life had truly begun.[7] "In the best Judeo-Christian tradition," she later said, "I believe that one must leave the world a better place than you found it."[8] The park would be just her first step in fulfilling that credo.

The Lauders had a wonderful partnership, due in part to a pact they had made when they married. Although corporate executives, they would never discuss business after hours. They could, however, set aside the pact in the mornings as they got ready for the workday. In the twenty minutes it took for Leonard to shower and shave and Evelyn to apply her makeup, they would chat about a shipment to I. Magnin or the introduction of a new fragrance at Saks Fifth Avenue. It got their business juices flowing. Consequently, when they purchased a ten-room co-op just off Fifth Avenue in June 1972, the design of the master bathroom was as important to them as the boardroom they had designed when the company became one of the first tenants in the new General Motors Building. Home and work were now just a few blocks apart, both with wonderful views of Central Park.

It had been thirty-two years since Evelyn had fled certain death at the hands of the Nazis. Now she was living a life she and her parents never could have imagined. At thirty-six, she was at the pinnacle of her career as corporate spokesperson. Her warm smile, vivacious personality, and natural beauty made journalists flock to her. And she was oh so quotable:

"I find that people are not clean enough. Really healthy skin is clean skin."[9]

"Who's got time at the end of the day to spend creaming her face for ages in front of a mirror?" (The answer was Estée Lauder's new "night table cream.")[10]

"With skirts going long, the face becomes more important and it needs vivid definition. So, we created lip tints of high-intensity glisten with low-intensity color."

"We've created products even a sensitive skin can use. They're made from pure skim milk."

She spoke the truth about it all. At an early age, her mother had begun teaching her about good skin care. After she "fell into the beauty business backwards," as she often said, it was easy to speak about the quality of the Estée Lauder products and the integrity of the company.[11]

It was all music to Leonard's ears. "The company and I grew up together," he was fond of saying, "our lives as closely paired as twins."[12] It was no surprise, then, when on December 12, 1972, it was announced that he would be ascending to the post of president of the company, although Estée would remain very much involved.

That same month, the average life span for a man in America was 67.4 years. Evelyn's father beat that statistic by nine years. Eisig (Ernst) Hausner, the man who had given everything to save his family, died at the end of December. He was seventy-six.

⁓

As June 1974 began in Montgomery County, Maryland, Rose was sending query letters to magazine and newspaper editors at a brisk clip, churning out articles on a variety of subjects. The Vietnam War was still a favorite, although she and Harvey weren't always on the same page. Harvey favored peace through strength. Rose favored peace through peace. When John Kerry had testified against the war before the Senate Committee on Foreign Relations three years earlier, she had taken thirteen-year-old Lesley to make her point.

Rose believed the more information she could absorb, the more articles she could write. And the more clips (published articles) she could collect, the better her chances of publishing with bigger fish. Most of her work was still appearing in Jewish papers. The *Baltimore Jewish Times* had accepted "The Palestinian

Question: What Nixon Should Know," a history lesson in religion and Middle East politics. It would run in the June 28, 1974, issue.

The *Jewish Week* editor agreed to publish Rose's article "Tay-Sachs an Issue in Abortion Hearings" in late June as well. Named for the two doctors who identified the disease, Tay-Sachs was a genetic disorder, resulting in the destruction of nerve cells in the brain and spinal cord. Infants born with it were severely disabled and typically died in their first years of life. Prenatal genetic testing could determine whether a fetus had inherited the defective gene that caused the condition. The parents would then have to wade through what must have been immeasurable grief in deciding whether or not to terminate the pregnancy. Rose felt a personal connection to the grieving families. Not only did the condition strike the Ashkenazi Jewish population at a disproportionate rate, but it no doubt brought back memories of her infant son's death from a congenital heart problem.

Two weeks before either of those pieces would appear, Rose was luxuriating in a bubble bath. It was a Saturday night, June 15, and she and Harvey had the house—and the television—to themselves. Gantt was now twenty-two and Todd was eighteen, both living on their own. Lesley was sixteen and out at a friend's house for the night. "Don't take too long," Harvey had called to Rose as she headed upstairs. "It's a great night to be home—Archie Bunker, *M*A*S*H*, and a Humphrey Bogart oldie!"[13]

Rose was shaving under her left arm when the little finger of her right hand brushed over a tiny bump at the edge of her left nipple. Fear froze her. Panicked thoughts swirled through her head. Despite all her other knowledge, Rose knew nothing about breast cancer. And all the women she knew who had ever been diagnosed with it had died: Harvey's cousin and two aunts (none of whom she had ever met), a friend, and friends of friends.

Washington, D.C.'s, most famous survivor, President Theodore Roosevelt's daughter, Alice Roosevelt Longsworth, was outspoken about her mastectomies (she had one in 1956 and another in 1970, when she was eighty-six), proclaiming afterward that she was the only topless octogenarian in town. But Rose only knew *of* Alice; she didn't actually *know* her. Besides, someone like Alice was a legend; mere mortal women like Rose died of breast cancer.

In that moment, Rose was at the same crossroads where nearly eighty thousand other women would find themselves in 1974: that of science and culture.[14] She would either die of a misunderstood disease or spend the rest of her life stripped of a breast—at a time when many in the United States thought breasts were the crown jewel of beauty and femininity.

⁓

Bosoms. Tatas. Knockers. Titties. No matter what you call them, breasts have been front and center throughout human history (pun intended). From Renaissance art to *Playboy* magazine covers (the magazine's tagline is "entertainment for men," also pun intended), society had long emphasized that breasts are the undeniable body structures that make women desirable. Many young women agonize over the timing of their breast development, and after their breasts develop, they agonize over their size, and later over their perkiness.

Portrayed in art with equal enthusiasm is the maternal breast, depicting the value of women as the nurturers of the species. Such is the breast's importance that science drew on the Latin word for breast, *mamilla,* to label the entire taxonomic class to which humans belong: mammals.

In the animal kingdom, a sense of smell is key for finding the best mates. In many species females give off scents (pheromones) to attract males and notify them of a readiness to mate. For humans, however, attraction is all about the sense of sight. Many studies reveal that men may notice a woman's face or hair, but it's her chest that most often draws their attention. And as the twentieth century went by, breasts became more visible with each year.

A voluptuous plastic bustline rocked the toy world on March 9, 1959, when Barbie debuted at the New York Toy Fair. Her Rubenesque chest (completely out of proportion to her tiny hips) worried toy buyers. Would mothers let their daughters play with dolls so overtly feminine, as opposed to the rather ungendered dolls of the era? Overwhelmingly, they did. And beginning a decade later, a number of those same little girls, now grown, brought their own breasts to the center of the women's movement, unleashing them by burning their bras.

A most notable bra-burning incident occurred in Atlantic City, New Jersey, just outside the venue of the 1968 Miss America pageant, an event famous for celebrating the contestants' figures. The article covering the protest went on to also include vital information on that year's winner: "Miss [Judith] Ford . . . is five-feet seven inches tall, 125 pounds and measures 36-24½-36."[15]

Women's magazines of the era were replete with articles about breasts and tantalizing advertisements for ways to enlarge smaller mammaries. The Princess Bust Developer was billed as a "new scientific help to nature." It was a toilet-plunger-type device that came with a jar of Bust Cream to rub on between plungings.[16]

Madame Du Barrie of Chicago guaranteed that her Positive French Method would grow a bustline by two to eight inches in just thirty days. The ad didn't describe just how the method worked, but if the small-busted customer included a two-cent stamp, Madame would send an illustrated booklet.[17]

Perhaps the most famous of all bust enhancers came from the Mark Eden company. One happy customer claimed that after "eight short weeks" she increased her bustline from 35½ inches to 39 inches.[18] Mark Eden's revolutionary bust developer was a pink plastic clamshell-like device with a spring in the middle that a woman squeezed between her hands. Ironically, the product exercised and strengthened the pectoralis major, the very muscle that Dr. Halsted and his protegés routinely removed with their radical mastectomies.

In the 1970s, more than 90 percent of medical school students were men.[19] In taking the Hippocratic oath at graduation, they vowed, "I will do no harm or injustice to them [patients]." Yet, despite the predominant male view that breasts were the ultimate symbol of beauty and maternity, breast surgeons (also predominantly male) were able to unceremoniously remove them when they became cancerous. The unfortunate aftermath was that their women patients who had bought into society's breast worship were left feeling grotesque and neutered.

⌐

"If my head pretended for a minute that nothing was there, my stomach knew immediately something was wrong," Rose later wrote. "It coiled into a tight ball and stayed that way for weeks."[20] The description of her physical reaction upon the discovery of a lump near her left nipple couldn't be more clear. Anyone ever faced with terror, cancer or otherwise, can relate to that gut-wrenching sensation.

Harvey came into the bathroom to tell her that dinner was ready and it was just about time for Archie Bunker. "Feel this place," she instructed him. He followed her orders but didn't find anything. She handed him the soap. "Try feeling the place with soap on your finger."[21]

He did. "There's something there," he said, nodding slightly.

They went through the rest of the weekend mechanically. But as soon as Monday rolled around, Rose became a hurricane of activity. She started dialing the office of her internist, Dr. Bernard Heckman, long before it actually opened at nine. Rose's was the first call the receptionist took.

"I found a lump in my left breast," Rose told her. The receptionist asked her to be there in an hour. How would Rose fill that hour? By calling Georgetown University Hospital, ten miles away. Rose had read about a thermography machine—a new breast cancer detection machine that used breast tissue temperature differences to detect cancer—that the hospital was installing. A few minutes later, she had an appointment for a thermogram for that Friday, June 21, at 10:00 a.m.

When Dr. Heckman examined her, he recommended a xeromammogram, another new type of X-ray, with results printed on paper as opposed to film; supposedly it made them easier to read. That machine was at another hospital just three miles away, and in minutes Rose had an appointment there for one o'clock that afternoon. Regardless of the xeromammogram results, Dr. Heckman told Rose, the lump still had to come out. He asked her if she had anyone in mind to do the biopsy.

"Just that I want a breast specialist," she answered. This surprised the doctor. "It's got to be an oncologist," she added firmly. (At the time, cancer surgeons and those who administered chemotherapy were one and the same, unlike today, with surgery as a separate specialty.)

The fact that she knew that word surprised him even more, and he asked her why she insisted on an oncologist who was also a breast specialist. Rose quipped, "If I had a detached retina, you'd send me to an optometrist, wouldn't you? Then why send me to a general surgeon for cancer?"[22]

To that he had no answer, nor was he aware of anyone to refer her to. But he was happy to sign a referral letter to take with her. At the hospital for her xeromammogram, she asked how long it would take before the results were ready. The technician said Dr. Heckman should have them the next morning. Rose's last stop of the day was the public library. A card catalogue search on the term "breast cancer" disappointingly produced just one book, which she checked out.

Rose knew there was a breast cancer clinic at the National Institutes of Health (NIH), just three miles away, and she called to make an appointment. NIH was also home to the National Library of Medicine, the largest collection of medical literature in the world. She reasoned that since she lived so close, she might as well take advantage of it. She was at its door when it opened the next morning.

Every document and book Rose scanned confirmed Dr. Heckman's advice. The lump had to be removed. Mammograms, she learned, were accurate 85 percent of the time. That nugget of information hit home when she paused her reading to call Dr. Heckman's office about the results and the nurse told her, "Everything's fine." Given her recent research, the nurse's response didn't ignite much confidence. What if she was in that other, "non-fine" 15 percent? A biopsy would be the only sure way to know the lump wasn't malignant.

Most surgeons removed the entire lump and sent it off to pathology while the patient was still unconscious. If there was no cancer, the patient went home. But if the pathology showed cancer, a radical mastectomy was performed on the spot. Sometimes the doctor came out to the waiting room to advise the patient's family in advance; sometimes not. Why should a woman's doctor, husband, father, or brother, or anyone else, decide for her? Rose wondered.

Certainly, there were women for whom a second trip to the operating room would pose a high risk (women who had certain types of other health conditions, for example). The so-called one-step procedure might make sense for them. But Rose could think of no other grounds for a woman not to have a voice in her own treatment, which would mean some time between the biopsy and any subsequent surgery. The more she read, the more she was convinced.

One of the most compelling reasons was the psychological factor. "Needing a mastectomy would be bad enough," she thought, "but not having time to adjust to the idea in advance seemed absolutely barbaric."[23]

In addition, Rose reasoned, extra time would allow a woman to do research on the disease. Just three days earlier, she had been a living example of most women's blissful ignorance about breast cancer. She was a skilled researcher, however, having honed that proficiency over nearly thirty years, beginning with her days in Dr. Gantt's lab. Other women most likely would not have had that experience, nor would they have the luxury of living practically on top of the National Library of Medicine. Lastly, with a two-step procedure, a woman could take her time selecting a surgeon. And it appeared as though that selection would be life-altering.

Surgeon-turned-author Dr. George Crile Jr. would have agreed with all of Rose's reasoning. His was the single book that she had found in the public library the day before. Published a year earlier, it was titled *What Women Should Know About the Breast Cancer Controversy*. Of course, Rose had no idea there even was a controversy.[24] But she was about to learn a great deal more in a very short amount of time.

⌁

Dr. George Washington Crile Jr. would eventually become one of the heroes of modern breast cancer treatment. It would be a long and difficult road, however. Dr. Crile had grown up in medicine. His father, Dr. George Crile Sr., was a founder of the Cleveland Clinic and had made important contributions to the study of blood pressure. The younger Dr. Crile spent all his time at the Cleveland Clinic, with the exception of his World War II service from 1942 to 1946—an experience that changed the course of his career.

Researching service members' ruptured appendixes, he discovered they were not as life-threatening as previously thought. If patients were given anti-infection drugs and transported to a full-service hospital for the surgery, they had a much better outcome than if they were treated in the field. "I came home from World War II convinced that operations in many fields of surgery were either too radical, or not even necessary," Dr. Crile later said.[25] This was revolutionary enough, but when he turned his attention to the treatment of cancer, he really rattled the cages of his fellow doctors.

The book that Rose had found in her library was Dr. Crile's third on the subject of cancer. His first, *Cancer and Common Sense,* was released on November 4, 1955. (That was the book Shirley had read before her biopsy and mastectomy.) On October 31, in advance of the book's release, Dr. Crile wrote a multipage article for *Life* magazine. He began his piece with an anecdote about a seventy-five-year-old woman he had just met. She was paralyzed and unable to speak. Her family physician had found a lump in her thyroid gland and surmised that a cancerous tumor was preventing her speech. He further postulated that it had metastasized to her brain, causing the paralysis. And then he referred her to Dr. Crile.

X-rays were taken and a series of tests run, while the woman remained stuporous in her hospital bed. Dr. Crile found no cancer. When he spoke to the woman's son and two daughters, he explained, "There's nothing that can be done. Your mother has suffered a stroke from a broken blood vessel, her brain is irreparably damaged. There is no operation or treatment that can help her in any way."

The older daughter's voice quavered as she asked, "Did you find cancer?" Dr. Crile replied that he had not. "Thank God," the three siblings proclaimed together. The doctor was shocked, even more so when he realized their rationale. Had there been cancer, he knew the woman might have had a chance of it being "cured" (the magic word of the time), whereas the hemorrhage could not be cured. Yet the family was more frightened of cancer than of their mother's actual terminal condition.[26]

Dr. Crile's lengthy treatise went on to explain that cancer wasn't a single disease but a large family of diseases, related only in name. It was no harder to live with, or die from, than any other disease, he pointed out. But he had other concerns. "Those responsible for telling the public about cancer have chosen to use the weapon of fear," he wrote, "believing that only through fear can the public be educated."

Be vigilant or you will die instantly was the common message. The public listened, insisting on superfluous tests, unnecessary operations, and the consequent undue psychological distress.

"The advocates of early diagnosis are not wrong," Dr. Crile said. "They have merely overemphasized their point." Even when cancer was confirmed and surgery was recommended, fear pushed some people to demand it immediately. It was precisely that rush that Dr. Mayo had urged in his quote for Samuel Adams's 1913 *Ladies Home Journal* article. Dr. Crile eloquently advised, "You have time in which to think. A week or even a month will probably make no difference. Do not panic."[27]

By this time Dr. Crile was considered a medical maverick, and his critics were many. Physician representatives of the American Medical Association, the National Cancer Institute, the American Cancer Society, and the country's leading cancer hospitals labeled him as dangerous and fatalistic. They were especially critical of his stance on breast cancer. While Dr. Crile pointed out that the well-done, conservative operations (those that left unaffected lymph nodes, muscles, and bones intact) then being performed in Scotland and other European countries were as effective as a radical mastectomy, the Halsted disciples were insistent in their rebukes of him.

Dr. Crile admitted to having performed radical surgeries. He pointed out that only by doing so did he and other surgeons with similar beliefs learn about the limits of such procedures. By the time he wrote *What Women Should Know About the Breast Cancer Controversy* in 1973, not only was he hoping that surgeons would move away from the Halsted approach, but he had also become a fan of a new type of breast surgery: the lumpectomy. It took only the tumor and some surrounding tissue, leaving the breast intact. He was against axillary lymph node removal, which interrupted the lymph system's essential purpose. (Today's sentinel node biopsy wouldn't become the standard until the beginning of the twenty-first century.)

Dr. Crile's last point regarding the breast cancer controversy involved the idea of putting a woman through the trauma of removing a breast when the cancer had already spread to her lungs or brain or bones. He believed it was just plain cruel. And he had personal knowledge of that fact. In 1958, between his two books, his wife, Jane, was diagnosed with metastatic breast cancer. She dutifully had a mastectomy, yet died five years later, at the age of fifty-four.

Even after retirement, he stood firm in his beliefs, stating, "Universal acceptance of a procedure does not necessarily make it right."

Dr. Crile and Rose had never met. Via his writing, however, he talked her out of hoping for a lumpectomy: "Cancers that are large in relation to the size of the breast, cancers that are located near the center of the breast . . . are *not* well adapted to treatment by partial mastectomy."[28] Rose's unwelcome lump bordered her nipple. His book also taught her about partial and modified mastectomies, the infamous Halsteds, and breast reconstruction; she tucked away the information about the last until after her recovery.

The statistics showed that 90 percent of American surgeons performed Halsted mastectomies.[29] Yet in all the reading Rose had done, not a single cancer expert mentioned that removing the pectoral muscle was necessary. Consequently, she was determined that hers would remain securely in place.

When Friday, June 21, rolled around, Rose had her thermogram at Georgetown University Hospital and then went to her appointment at the NIH breast center. The doctor examined her and explained that in order to be treated there, the protocol called for a series of tests to be done first. Rose protested at the amount of time that would take, and the doctor nodded in agreement. "If it were my wife, I'd tell her to have the tumor biopsied immediately."[30] She asked for referrals to doctors in private practice she could contact, and he gave her a list.

Rose dressed and changed a couple of dollar bills into nickels and dimes for the phone booth (calls were fifteen cents each). Dialing each number on her list, she explained to the doctor on the other end that she was seeking a two-step procedure. She was met with absolute wrath.

"No patient is going to tell me how to do my surgery."

"I've never heard of such a thing."

"You're absolutely ridiculous!"

"If the diagnosis is positive on frozen section [in the pathology lab in the middle of her surgery], the breast must come off immediately."[31]

Rose was living through Dr. Crile's controversy, as well as the backlash he had faced. In frustration, she called Dr. Heckman. If it was just a biopsy she wanted, he suggested, why not go to the general surgeon who had done Harvey's hernia? Rose followed that advice, meeting the doctor long after his regular office hours had ended. After an exam, he agreed to do the biopsy and called the hospital to schedule it for Tuesday, June 25.

The next day, June 22, was Rose's forty-third birthday. A biopsy with no mastectomy attached would have been the best gift she could have hoped for. Although her "streak of stubbornness and a loud voice," as she would later say, weren't bad gifts either.[32]

The surgeon who would be doing the biopsy had stitched up many of the Kushner children's cuts along with Harvey's hernia. Still, Rose wasn't taking any chances. With a lawyer's help, she had crafted a document to be signed prior to her going into the operating room: "Under no circumstances is [a blank to fill in the doctor's name] or anyone else in the operating room of [a blank for the hospital] to perform the procedure known as mastectomy (removal of either breast). I hereby release [another blank for the doctor] and all other parties connected with the above consented-to procedure from any liability for damage sustained by me due to my refusal to consent to the procedure known as mastectomy (removal of either breast)."[33]

When she checked into the hospital the next day, she drew scribbles over any lines on the admission form giving the doctor blanket permission to do "anything deemed necessary." She also refused disposal of "the tissue removed," figuring she'd take it with her to whoever agreed to her mastectomy terms. The surgeon patronizingly signed the form, making light of it. He was absolutely certain nothing dark was lurking in Rose's chest.

When she came to, his face drifted into view. "I've got bad news," he said sharply. "It's cancer." Then he turned on his heel and left. One of the nurses patted Rose's hand, explaining she had hurt his feelings by not allowing him to finish the job. Rose nodded and mumbled, "I know. But for cancer I want more than a general surgeon."

"I'd do the same thing in your shoes, Mrs. Kushner," the nurse said. "Exactly the same."[34]

Rose would be spending the night at the hospital, but she and Harvey had begun making plans earlier in the afternoon. Since she hadn't agreed to enter the protocol at NIH, being treated there was now out of the question. However, after a call to a friend there, Rose had an appointment with a breast cancer specialist at New York City's Memorial Sloan Kettering Cancer Center (MSKCC). She would see him the next afternoon. When Harvey picked her up at the hospital on Wednesday morning, Rose was ready for the two-hundred-mile trip north, clutching her pathology slides and the jar with her pickled tumor.

The New York physician explained his surgical technique in a soft monotone. Still not thinking clearly because of the lingering effects of the anesthesia the previous day, Rose caught only a few words: "incision . . . axillary nodes . . . pectoral muscles . . . some permanent disability." He never uttered the words "Halsted radical." But it all became clearer after a few sips of Scotch back in their hotel room.

"He wants to do a Halsted," she told Harvey. "That's what he meant. It didn't sink in."[35] Harvey started making calls, eventually reaching a business associate at his firm's New York office. That person recommended a doctor at Roswell Park Cancer Center in Buffalo. It was a state hospital and had the distinction of being the first institution in the world to focus exclusively on cancer research. And it was a hospital that *no longer* performed *any* Halsteds. The Kushners flew the three hundred miles to Buffalo that night.

When Dr. Thomas Dao came into the examination room the next morning, his warm smile and floppy polka-dot tie immediately put Rose at ease. Dr. Dao was born on April 27, 1921, in Suzhou, China, making him only eight years her senior. Yet his calm demeanor gave him an aura of aged wisdom. Most impressive of all, as the director of the breast surgery department at Roswell since 1957, his research had guided him down the same path that Dr. Crile had taken. Dr. Dao explained that no studies showed superior patient outcomes with Halsted radical mastectomies. So why do them? Why permanently cripple women just because it had always been done that way? And like Dr. Crile, he also had many detractors.

After her exam, Dr. Dao ordered two days' worth of X-rays and blood tests for Rose. When Saturday morning rolled around, he told her he would schedule her for a modified radical mastectomy the following Tuesday, July 2. As crazy as it seemed, Rose was thrilled and triumphant. Her pectoral muscles and lymph nodes wouldn't be touched. Still-better news came once the surgery was over. Dr. Dao told Rose all of the cancer had been removed with the biopsy. Plus, the lymph nodes he had tested were clear of cancer. After seventeen days of worry, she was finally able to relax.

Because she was so far from home, Dr. Dao kept her at Roswell longer than the customary seven to ten days. She was there for three weeks, just to make certain she was healing properly and without complications. Just a few days post-surgery, however, and long before she went home, Rose began scribbling notes, mainly in the form of questions. Why wasn't the medical profession more open to two-step procedures? What was driving the cruel one-step status quo? Why were other patients not insistent about being involved in their breast cancer treatment? Why were women not given the freedom of choice? It was the last one that was the biggie.

The day Dr. Dao came in to take off Rose's bandages—telling her she could now wear a loose bra with absorbent cotton stuffed into the empty cup—would have been a big deal on its own. But he enhanced that celebration by inviting her to visit his endocrine research lab. Given that Roswell was a research hospital and her surgeon was a well-respected researcher, research junkie Rose felt like she had just hit it big on a Las Vegas slot machine. Everything she saw in the lab prompted questions, which Dr. Dao answered, not as if she were just a patient, but as if she were the medical reporter she had been before cancer had intervened in her life.

There was no question in Rose's mind that writing an article about her experience with breast cancer would be the first project she undertook as soon as she was home. Between what she already knew and what she could learn at NIH and the Library of Medicine, it would be just what the doctor ordered for American women.

Rose had always prided herself on accurate reporting. But on that Saturday evening in the bath when her mind had searched for names of other women who had had breast cancer and Alice Roosevelt Longworth popped into her head, Rose assumed she'd survived because of her rarified status. But women of a similar status didn't always survive.

On October 8, 1811, in an operation that took less than thirty minutes, famed Boston surgeon John Warren amputated Abigail "Nabby" Adams Smith's right breast. She was the daughter of John Adams, America's second president (and the sister of John Quincy Adams, who would be the sixth president). She was tied down to a bed in her parents' home and the surgery was performed without anesthesia; Nabby was given a cloth-wrapped stick to bite on when the pain overwhelmed her (how could it not have?). It took another hour for Dr. Warren and his assistants to stop the bleeding, cauterizing the tissue with a hot iron spatula. Less than two years later, Nabby died of metastasized disease.[36]

Breast cancer had touched another American president decades earlier. George Washington's mother, Mary, had found a lump but delayed having her breast examined, perhaps because of the savage nature of mastectomies of that era. By the time she did seek medical help, the cancer had spread too far for surgery, and she succumbed to it in 1789, just four months after her son became the first American president.[37]

Cancer had also touched royalty. Anne of Austria became the queen of France in 1615, marrying Louis XIII. Twenty-two years later the queen (at the advanced age of thirty-six) gave birth to her first child, the boy who would be-come Louis XIV five years later. Stories of the boy king abound. His was the longest reign in French history (seventy-two years), filled with lavish parties and the grand construction of his summer home, the chateau of Versailles. But he was powerless against his mother's breast cancer. Anne discovered a lump in 1663 and, fearing the horrific cancer treatments of the time, ignored it. When her breast became hardened from tumors, she finally consented to topical treat-ments. It was too late for her as well; she died in 1666 at the age of sixty-four.[38]

Cancer has never been particular about whom it strikes: rich or poor, pow-erful or meek, good or evil. For centuries it was handled in silence in nearly all cases. It was because of that silence that Rose found so little information on breast cancer. She, however, would not be silent. The breast cancer crusade was about to go public in a big way.

Chapter 6

The President Has Made His Decision

Four years before Rose's mastectomy, on the frosty morning of January 14, 1970, Democratic senator Gaylord Nelson and his lead staffer, Ben Gordon, were walking from their office to the Capitol. A group of women on the Capitol steps shouted at them, the condensation from their breath hanging in the air like fire from dragons. This was only the beginning of the day for Senator Nelson. The story, however, started centuries before.

Women, and their male lovers, had long sought methods to prevent pregnancy. Ancient Egyptian women inserted a mixture of honey, acacia leaves, and lint into their vaginas to block sperm. As time passed, other solutions were found, including sea sponges and lemon halves, leading the way to the first condom: a linen sheath tied with a ribbon. Centuries later, the linen was replaced with vulcanized rubber.[1]

And then the world met the anti-pornography king, Anthony Comstock. An 1873 U.S. law bearing his name forbade the distribution of contraceptive devices and information. Comstock opined that contraception was "obscene, lewd, lascivious, filthy, indecent and disgusting."[2] The penalty for breaking that law was five years in jail. Consequently, many women turned to abortions to terminate unwanted pregnancies. Some survived the often barbaric and unclean surgical procedures; others did not.

By the time World War II ended—researchers having produced a number of valuable pharmaceuticals to help the military effort during that conflict— scientists turned their attention to the creation of an oral contraceptive (OC). Imagine the excitement on June 23, 1960, when G. D. Searle and Company released Enovid, the first birth control pill to hit the market. Enovid's developers promoted its additional benefits, stating that it "corrected menstrual disorders" and was a preventive against breast cancer. "Not one woman of eight hundred who took birth control pills over a five year period developed cancer of the breast," co-creator Dr. Gregory Pincus proclaimed triumphantly. He added that OCs should actually be considered "health pills."[3] That would get them around any twentieth-century Comstocks who might be lurking in the shadows.

Sales began growing. By 1965, one out of every four married American women under the age of forty-five had used "the Pill," its new moniker. (Unmarried women couldn't procure it until 1972.) By 1967, nearly thirteen million women were using the Pill worldwide.[4] The women's movement, the women's health movement, and Betty Friedan's NOW had been clear in their belief that women could never be free to have educations and careers if they continued having unplanned pregnancies. OCs would now give women that freedom, becoming— aside from penicillin—"the century's most revolutionary medical breakthrough."[5]

However, freedom isn't free, as the saying goes. As time passed, women on the Pill began seeing their doctors for an assortment of maladies, including breast tenderness, weight gain, and dizziness. Some also developed migraines, uterine fibroids, and high blood pressure. The first unfavorable reports linking these conditions to the Pill were downplayed by doctors, women, and the pharmaceutical companies. Then rumblings of potential links between cancer and the Pill were heard. And when an alarming number of women developed blood clots (thromboembolic disease), women became justifiably anxious.

One of these was Barbara Seaman, a medical journalist and doctor's wife. She masterfully laid out the concerning issues in her November 1969 book, *The Doctors' Case Against the Pill.* Not only did her researched prose deliver a gut punch, but a cast of well-respected doctors went on record with their concerns as well.

"The Pill allows experiments on the general population that would never be allowed as a planned experiment," one wrote.

Another said, "Never in history have so many individuals confidently consumed such a powerful medication with so little information as to potential hazards."[6]

The doctors' testimonies, added to those of women who had taken the Pill, built a case against its safety. But the book didn't spark the national outrage Barbara had hoped for. Then she read about the hearings Senator Nelson was convening. He was chair of the Subcommittee on Monopoly, a part of the Select Committee on Small Business. His hearings, "Competitive Problems in the Drug Industry," would investigate abuses in the use of antibiotics, barbiturates, and tranquilizers.

Barbara sent the senator a six-page letter outlining her book and her concerns. Nelson passed the letter to Gordon, who did research on the issue and recommended adding birth control pills to the hearing. There hadn't been widely publicized notice of the hearings, so Nelson and Gordon hadn't expected to see those members of D.C. Women's Liberation outside the Capitol that morning. Nor did they realize there was another contingent of the group waiting in the gallery of the stately hearing room.

As the morning progressed, the physician witnesses spoke of the disconcerting side effects of the Pill. Alice Wolfson and her sisters in D.C. Women's Liberation sat quietly, becoming more and more outraged that their doctors had never discussed any of the risks now being presented. Nor could they believe that not a single woman was testifying that day. Although there would be several women physicians heard by the subcommittee in ensuing days, no patients were ever called.

Among those testifying in support of the Pill was Columbia professor and obstetrics specialist Dr. Elizabeth Connell. She wasted no words in her warning that if women were made aware of the Pill's hazards, they'd give up contraception entirely, producing unwanted children she called "Nelson babies."[7] Unfortunately for the senator, the press would reprint that phrase hundreds of times.

The consensus thus far was that the Pill's side effects were caused by its high concentration of synthetic estrogens. Dr. Roy Hertz, of Rockefeller University, was asked if the Pills caused cancer. He said no, but finished the sentence with something even more poignant: "They are to breast cancer what fertilizer is to the wheat crop." In other words, if cancer was a seed, the estrogen in the Pill would fuel its growth.[8]

At this, Wolfson jumped up. "We are not going to sit quietly any longer," she shouted. "You're murdering us for your profit and convenience." She demanded that women who had taken the Pill be allowed to testify. A shocked Senator Nelson replied, "We're not going to let these proceedings be interrupted in this way. If you ladies would sit down—"

But Wolfson cut him off. "Our lives have been interrupted by taking this pill!"

She, and all of those with her, had experienced one or more of the side effects that were finally coming to light. Wolfson said afterward in an interview, "We will no longer tolerate intimidation by white-coated gods, antiseptically directing our lives."[9]

The hearings were scheduled for four more days. On the last day, Dr. Philip Coffman of the NIH uttered the most frightening words of all: "Indeed, there appears to be no organ system tested that is not affected [by the Pill and its estrogen] in some way. With such comprehensive involvement, who knows, or can intelligently estimate, what the risks are?"[10]

The Pill hearings would go on to be the longest-running congressional hearings in American history, lasting over a decade. They became known as "the Boston Tea Party of the women's health movement."[11] But there was still a long way to go in changing women's health in America.

⁓

"Writers write. Everything is a story." Rose's own words resonated in her head throughout her recuperation in Buffalo. How could it be, she kept asking herself, that, in a year as enlightened as 1974, and in a nation as mighty in all forms of science as the United States of America, there was so little written about breast cancer specifically for the patients themselves? Like Shirley Temple Black nearly two years earlier, Rose felt compelled, or more accurately *driven,* to help the millions of other women who would follow her with the same diagnosis.

Even before she returned home at the end of July, Rose was busily conceiving a series of magazine and newspaper articles. Then it hit her: she was thinking too small. While articles would be great support vehicles, they would be too scattered across publications and time frames for desperate women to hunt down. She needed to write a book, a digestible encyclopedia that would take women from detection through treatment to recovery.

It wouldn't be a memoir. Rose had recently read one published two years earlier called *The Invisible Worm,* by *Seventeen* magazine editor Babette Rosmond. She wrote under the pseudonym Rosamond Campion and, coincidentally, had been treated by Dr. George Crile, whose identity she also omitted. Rose thought the cloak-and-dagger of hiding behind a pseudonym was ridiculous. As all the experts had told her, the number-one reason women hesitate to have lumps checked is fear. What help was a book by a breast cancer survivor whose author was afraid to use her own name? Rose would use not only her name but her personal story as well to encourage women to go to a doctor, while also educating them about breast cancer and its treatment.

Once she was home and reconnected with her typewriter, query letters to newspaper, magazine, and book editors flew out like bees from a hive. In them, Rose explained that she had been appalled at how misinformed most "know-it-all family doctors" were. While she acknowledged she couldn't write for the medical profession, her hope was to get information to them by educating their female patients. She made it clear that she was not in agreement with the "women's lib" argument that mastectomies were being done unnecessarily.[12] Nor did she think any type of "male chauvinist pig" conspiracy was occurring, pointing out that prostate cancer treatment was in no better shape than that for breast cancer.[13] (For that matter, the small number of men who were diagnosed with breast cancer each year were completely ignored.) Rather, it was a simple case of the patients themselves not being aware of their growing options.

Options. That word resonated with Rose. The issue of giving women birth control options had drawn her to the press coverage of Nelson's Pill hearings back in 1970, and she wanted to know more than what the newspapers were printing. Her neighbor around the corner, Carrie Nelson, was happy to oblige, providing Rose with a transcript after the first round of hearings had ended on Capitol Hill. Carrie was Mrs. Gaylord Nelson. And while they were Wisconsin residents, the Nelsons also kept a Washington-area home, a common practice for members of Congress. Reading about the pharmaceutical companies' deception, the paltry number of women testifying, the terrifying link between too much estrogen and cancer, and the lack of information available for the patients had disturbed Rose in 1970. Now, with her experiences and what she'd learned since, that lack of information infuriated her.

Rose was a cigarette smoker, as were more than twenty million other American women in 1974. Breast cancer was not on the list of potential health risks of the habit. But every time Rose lit up, she saw the warning on the packet: "The Surgeon General Has Determined That Cigarette Smoking Is Dangerous to Your Health." Rose knew the risk before she struck the match.

Yet, given the ever-growing body of evidence of their connection to blood clots and breast cancer, not a single warning accompanied the Pill—not a label or a pamphlet. There was no question in Rose's mind that this topic would be a chapter in her book as well.

She had sent letters to publishers Macmillan and Random House about her book but got no response. The *New York Times* didn't respond to her query, either. A *Washington Post* editor thought maybe the paper could find a spot for an article in its Sunday supplement about giving treatment options to women diagnosed with breast cancer. Rose refused, telling him if it wasn't going in the main paper with its large readership, she wanted it back. He said he'd think about it. He would ultimately be back in touch with her sooner than he thought.

—

Like a sand castle built too close to the waves, President Richard Nixon's world was slowly eroding. It had begun the night of June 17, 1972, when a bumbling group of burglars had been nabbed at the Democratic Party headquarters in the Watergate office building. All pled not guilty, but as time passed, their pleas changed. The press and the public began asking questions about their motives and their unidentified boss. In the middle of it all, and unrelated to Watergate, Vice President Spiro Agnew resigned in October 1973 after a series of bribery allegations.

President Nixon's choice for a replacement was Michigan representative Gerald Ford. While Ford had thought Congress would be his last political position, he was happy to be sworn into office that December. But while Agnew's scandal had gone away, Watergate would not. Damaging testimony from the accused burglars, and even more damaging White House tape recordings, were eventually followed by fifty-one days of testimony before the Senate. Nixon was given two choices: be impeached (and most assuredly be convicted and removed from office) or resign.

Two weeks after Rose returned home from Buffalo, on August 8, 1974, at 9:01 p.m., Richard Nixon announced to the nation that he was resigning. Suddenly, just eight months after becoming vice president, Gerald Ford was president of the United States. Later that month, he nominated former New York governor Nelson Rockefeller as his vice president. That whirlwind of events, however, was not the most dramatic of 1974 for the Fords or the Rockefellers.

Thursday, September 26, was a lovely fall day. Nancy Howe, personal assistant and friend to the First Lady, was headed to Bethesda Naval Hospital, near the National Institutes of Health. She had an appointment for a routine checkup, and since Mrs. Ford was due for her six-month checkup, Nancy encouraged the First Lady to come along. During Mrs. Ford's exam, the doctor checked her breasts and then excused himself. When he returned, he was accompanied by a surgeon. After another breast exam, Mrs. Ford dressed and returned to the White House. There she found a note that the First Family's doctor wanted to see her and the president. When they met that evening, the doctor explained that a suspicious lump had been identified in Mrs. Ford's right breast. It had to come out immediately.[14]

The Bethesda operating rooms were occupied throughout the next day, so her surgery was scheduled for Saturday morning. The First Lady arrived at the hospital at six Friday evening and was checked into the Presidential Suite. The secure and autonomous cluster of rooms, including a sitting room, kitchen, conference room, hospital bedroom, and office, wasn't terribly high up in the twenty-story building. Consequently, Mrs. Ford and her family, who had joined her for dinner, had a bird's-eye view of what was happening below. Tipped off that presidential limousines had arrived, a gaggle of press was forming. Their stories would fill the Saturday morning papers.[15]

Rose lived literally five minutes from the hospital. Like the press, she knew tipsters, too. She didn't need to wait for the newspapers to figure out the story. "The stage was just being set too elaborately," she later said.[16] Desperate to speak with someone—anyone—who could help her prevent "a rush-railroading to a radical" on Mrs. Ford, Rose called Alice Roosevelt Longworth and other friends of the president whom she knew. No one was home. Finally, at 11:45 p.m., through a mutual friend, she reached presidential speechwriter Milton Friedman. Rose laid out all her reasons for Mrs. Ford to agree to a biopsy *only* the following morning. "The president should not let a general surgeon do the operation," she told him. "If the president's wife isn't going to get the best, who is?"[17]

Friedman heard her out and then said, "Just a minute, I'll see what I can do." When he returned, he said, "I am sorry, Mrs. Kushner. But the president has made his decision."

Rose was flabbergasted. "It's not his decision to make. Mrs. Ford should make that decision, don't you think?" Now Friedman was shocked. He repeated his words, adding that that was all he was authorized to say.[18]

The next morning, Bethesda's chief of surgery, forty-six-year-old Dr. William Fouty, arrived at the hospital. He was a Navy surgeon who had operated on Ford's knee a few years earlier, when he was a congressman. Dr. Fouty was assigned the task of deciding which way Mrs. Ford's one-step breast surgery would go. He could do a lumpectomy, but that was such an unknown procedure that he probably never entertained the possibility. He could go the modified radical mastectomy route, done more often than lumpectomies, but still not supported by enough solid evidence that it "cured" a patient. Or Dr. Fouty could take the safe road, the road 95 percent of all surgeons took when dealing with potential breast cancer, and the road he ultimately chose.[19] Once the tumor had been removed and examined in the pathology lab, Dr. Fouty performed a radical mastectomy, amputating Mrs. Ford's right breast, along with the underlying muscles and all of the lymph nodes under her arm.

The press coverage ran the gamut, including that Mrs. Ford had worn a "pink, quilted housecoat" for the dinner with her family the night before the surgery.[20] Journalists were careful, however, in their word choice about her potentially having cancer. She was in the hospital for an "exam" or an "exploratory surgery." She had a "nodule," which if "malignant" would be a bad thing. Some used the word *cancer* in the headline or first line only. A few used it more than once in their articles. Some didn't use it at all.

Rose and Harvey listened to the news coverage on the radio. When the broadcast finished, Harvey said to her, "Well, it looks like the wife of Harvey Kushner got a hell of a lot better treatment that the wife of Gerald Ford."[21]

Sunday morning's papers reported that Dr. Fouty proclaimed he was "cautiously optimistic" and that Mrs. Ford's surgery of nearly four hours went "exceedingly well." A cancerous tumor measuring less than an inch had been removed from her right breast, and he had seen no evidence of disease in the surrounding muscle or tissue. The doctor said a "standard radical mastectomy" was performed nonetheless.[22]

Rose read the articles like all other Americans were doing that morning. But her perspective was far different. She knew from her research there was no reason to do the biopsy and mastectomy in one step. There was no reason for the extensive, crippling surgery, leaving the functionality of Mrs. Ford's arm compromised the rest of her life. Furthermore, there was nothing "standard" about a woman (First Lady or not) losing a breast.

In 1957, a major general invited Dr. Bernard Fisher to a meeting on the subject of breast cancer. The invitation wasn't from just any general; this one had served admirably in the Pacific Theater during World War II and had operated on President Dwight Eisenhower. At the time, Dr. Fisher was happily working on liver regeneration. Breast cancer was not in his wheelhouse. Out of courtesy to the esteemed general, however, he went to the meeting, a move that ultimately would elevate breast cancer treatment out of Halsted's nineteenth century.

The meeting agenda included a conversation about tumor metastasis. That piqued Dr. Fisher's interest. But what sealed the deal in rerouting his career was the discussion of a newly established manner for collecting information: clinical trials, which had been conceived of only ten years earlier. The idea was that researchers could study a specific number of patients over a specific length of time, and under specific conditions to provide data on the effectiveness of a medical treatment—in this case, breast cancer surgery.

No one disagreed about the efficacy of surgery in treating breast cancer. The problem was the extent of that surgery, the very thing Rose had taken issue with. Dr. Fisher was always quick to acknowledge that Halsted had developed his mastectomy techniques based on the knowledge of his time. Fifty years later, it was common knowledge that cancer cells did not spread in the way Halsted had thought. They increased in the same way compounding interest did, and they traveled through the bloodstream, not just the lymphatic system.[23] While Dr. Fisher gave Halsted a pass for his misapprehensions, he was vocal in his belief that endorsing a procedure founded on Halsted's out-of-date principles was "irrational."

Like his contemporary Dr. Crile, Dr. Fisher was a strong advocate of less can be more. But no rigidly controlled clinical trials had ever been done to prove it. To that end, the National Cancer Institute convened a Breast Cancer Study Group in 1965. As if exploring an unknown galaxy, the doctors in the group organized areas of study (which would include the much-needed surgical trials) with the end goal of creating a coordinated breast cancer treatment program.

The study group was renamed the Breast Cancer Task Force in 1966. Dr. Fisher, Thomas Dao (Rose's surgeon), and many other cancer luminaries lent their time and talent to the task force, which presented its work to the scientific community each year. The 1974 presentation—entitled "Breast Cancer: Report to the Profession"—was scheduled for Monday, September 30. The report would deliver the findings of a study they had begun in 1971. With seventeen hundred women and thirty-seven hospitals, the study's purpose was to answer the question "Is the radical mastectomy—hardly changed over the previous one hundred years—the only option for breast cancer treatment?"[24]

Dr. Nate Berlin was the chair of the task force and had been planning this event for months. He worried that it wouldn't receive much public attention, even though 400 of the 488 seats in NIH's Masur Auditorium would be filled by breast cancer experts from around the world. Dr. Berlin needn't have fretted. Coming two days after Betty Ford's mastectomy, not only was the auditorium full, but it was an absolute media circus.[25]

The study in question showed that mastectomy, followed by "powerful anti-cancer drugs [chemotherapy] appear to stop the spread of breast cancer in high-risk cases."[26] Dr. Fisher was also on this task force and reported what would become the biggest news of all. After three years of follow-up, it appeared that there were no significant differences in the survival rates between Halsted radical mastectomies and the modified version, which left pectoral muscles intact.

The press became frenzied, linking that information to Mrs. Ford. Headlines screamed "Surgery Like First Lady's Might Offer No *Advantage*."[27]

Rose had planned to attend the presentation long before Mrs. Ford's cancer was announced. (In fact, the agenda she received when she arrived that fall morning would become the outline for her book.) She was thrilled to hear Dr. Fisher's astounding statement, boldly raising her left arm (something she could do because her muscles were intact after her mastectomy) and asking, "Is there ever any justification for excising [removing] the muscles?" "Only when there is evidence of invasion of the musculature," he answered. Rose asked how often that happened. Dr. Fisher replied, "Rarely."[28]

Across the street from the auditorium, Mrs. Ford was being closely monitored in her recovery. According to reports, her vitals were strong and her activities that day included raising her right hand to the top of her head (which she did without much difficulty despite having lost muscle), walking, sitting in a rocking chair, and lunching on tea, chicken broth, and crackers.[29] As with Shirley and Rose, Mrs. Ford's post-surgery thoughts began taking shape. She later said, "I lay in bed and watched television and saw on the news shows lines of women queued up to go in for breast examinations because of what happened to me."

It was phenomenal. The NCI saw inquiries about breast cancer shoot up, from their customary 250 per month to 2,500. Hospital switchboards across the county saw the same results. They had averaged twenty-five calls a day about the disease. Now they were receiving five hundred. It would later be reported that the number of women doing breast self-exams increased as well. Cancer researchers called the intense interest the "Betty Ford blip." The flood of women getting exams produced such a large number of suspicious lumps, hospital operating rooms were booked for months out.[30]

Mrs. Ford said she came to realize "the power of the woman in the White House. Not my power, but the power of the position, a power which could be used to help."[31]

The "Betty Ford blip" did more than save women's lives. It launched Rose into the stratosphere. The article about a woman's right to choose her breast cancer treatment that she had sent to the *Washington Post* back in August was suddenly very, *very* pertinent.[32] The editor scheduled it to run in the paper's main section Sunday, October 6, eight days after Mrs. Ford's surgery. The writing was masterful, and Rose's grasp of the medical information, along with the mastectomy controversy, was astounding for a woman who hadn't given cancer much thought six months earlier. Like Shirley Temple Black's hospital press conference, it was also groundbreaking. For the first time, a comprehensive article on breast cancer—at more than three thousand words—was running in one of the nation's most venerable papers. And for the first time, a breast cancer *survivor* gave a thorough account of her own experience.

In typical fashion, Rose joked to friends, "If I had known breast cancer would finally get me into the *Washington Post*, I'd have arranged to get it years ago!"[33] She also confided to Dr. Dao, "All this has changed my career from being a Jewish humorist to being a serious medical writer. Darn it! It was so much easier being funny!"[34]

Since the *Post* had put the article out on its wire service, hundreds of papers around the world picked it up. Rose felt bad that the article hadn't come out sooner; if it had, Mrs. Ford might have seen it and been more informed. However, the flip side of the coin, Rose observed, was that because of the sudden national focus on breast cancer, her words would probably now be more widely read. That, in turn, would help more women.

Helen Reddy's two-year-old hit song "I Am Woman, Hear Me Roar" was still a favorite, thanks to the fact that the women's movement had unofficially adopted it as their theme song. The lyrics of the refrain, "If I have to, I can do anything. I am strong, I am invincible," couldn't have been a better theme for Rose's belief about herself and the crusade she had launched.[35]

And she now occupied a much stronger position in book publishers' eyes. Harcourt Brace Jovanovich asked her to come to New York City at their expense on November 5. She nearly fainted when they presented her with a contract and a $10,000 advance (the equivalent of nearly $64,000 today).[36]

They agreed with her that visiting the hospitals of the European doctors she had heard speak at the NCI in September would be an excellent addition to her U.S. research and interviews. They were prepared to cover all of the expenses, plus those for visits to hospitals in Moscow and Leningrad. Rose would depart in three weeks, on Thanksgiving Day. After she left their offices, she mused that her current euphoria was 180 degrees from the terror she had experienced the last time she was in New York City, when death had hung over her like the sword of Damocles. What a ride it had been. And it was just beginning.

One of the women prompted by Betty Ford's surgery to do her own breast self-exam was Margaretta "Happy" Rockefeller, the wife of Nelson Rockefeller, the vice presidential appointee. She couldn't have been more shocked to discover a lump in her left breast on October 11, 1974. Six days later, she checked into MSKCC. Unlike the Halsted-aligned doctor Rose had met with, Mrs. Rockefeller was the patient of Dr. Jerome Urban, who performed a modified radical on her.[37]

Dr. Urban had stopped doing radicals a decade earlier after seeing a lack of evidence that they improved survival rates. At the same time, he began routinely taking a tissue sample from the corresponding position on the patient's other breast. A quick look at Mrs. Rockefeller's sample showed no cancer, but what remained of the tissue was still fixed in paraffin for more detailed examination the next day. To Dr. Urban's surprise, he saw a group of cancerous cells about the size of pinheads.[38]

Mrs. Rockefeller had just begun her recovery and was slightly anemic. Dr. Urban felt the physical and psychological burden of more surgery would be difficult. He did, however, tell her husband. They decided it would be best to withhold the information until just before the second surgery. (Keeping patients in the dark about their disease while informing relatives was an abhorrent, but not unusual, practice of the time.) Mrs. Rockefeller, however, asked the doctor about his biopsy findings, and Dr. Urban told her the truth.

For weeks, the women's sections of newspapers had been filled with the unbelievable story that, after all the country had been through in the preceding months, now both the First Lady *and* the future Second Lady had breast cancer. The Rockefellers visited the Fords in the White House in mid-November, and although the ladies discussed their surgeries with each other, Mrs. Rockefeller kept quiet about her pending second procedure.

The vice presidential couple were living amid turmoil. Rumors swirled about Nelson's infidelities, and because of his nomination, the Rockefellers' lives and bank accounts were being laid out in the nation's newspapers. Happy was a private person, often seen in New York alone, hiding behind large sunglasses. But Nelson seemed genuinely shaken by his wife's diagnoses. As he had done on the earlier occasion, his public announcement of the second surgery came the night before it occurred, on November 25. Again, American women wondered: would their breasts betray them, too?

~

"A slap in the face . . . an insult to Ghana . . . irrelevant and outrageous." Yale professor David Apter was regarded as the leading American authority on

Ghana in 1974. He was incensed when he heard the news that, on August 21, President Ford had appointed Shirley Temple Black as the new ambassador to the West African nation. Apter felt the post called for "a career foreign service officer or an experienced diplomat," and vowed to use the same ire when he sent a telegram of protest to Secretary of State Henry Kissinger.[39]

Shirley was accustomed to attacks like these, given her previous diplomatic appointments. Not only had her mastectomy not changed her interest in government affairs, but moving forward in that arena was a large part of her recovery. As soon as she was back in Washington in 1973, she had let President Nixon know she was ready for her next assignment. Given their friendship with the Nixons, the Blacks were invited to many important Washington events, including a black-tie state dinner honoring Soviet leader Leonid Brezhnev. That June 18 dinner had been highly publicized, sharing front-page space with the latest news on the Senate Watergate hearings.[40] Like many in America, Shirley had been shocked and saddened by the scandal and Nixon's ultimate resignation.

When the former U.S. ambassador to Ghana left his post in July 1974, replacing him was high on the incoming president's to-do list. Ghana had become independent from the United Kingdom in 1957. The nation of nearly ten million faced a multitude of challenges, including economic decline and emigration. Then came a coup d'état in 1966, resulting in the ouster of the elected prime minister and the installation of a military-led government.

Shirley was the first American woman ambassador to Ghana. Nonetheless, in many newspapers, the announcement of her new position appeared in the women's section, tucked between "fashion tips" and "helpful hints for homemakers." The photo frequently used in the piece was the same one that had been used in her *McCall's* breast cancer article two years earlier.

By the time of her appointment, breast cancer seemed a tiny blip in Shirley's very eventful life. Never one to look backward, preferring instead to embrace whatever the future held, Shirley felt she had done what she was called to do for her "sisters." The far-reaching impacts of her daring to rip away the veil of secrecy about the disease never occurred to her at the time. But it became an important part of her legacy. By turning her situation from that of a passive victim to a participant in all elements of her cancer treatment, Shirley had brought the women's health movement to breast cancer. And in so doing, she not only launched a national breast cancer dialogue; she also empowered women with two newly recognized tools.

The first came with her frank explanation of how she had discovered her breast lump. In 1972 breast self-exam (BSE) got little publicity, save for the American Cancer Society's newspaper ads for a BSE booklet they would send upon request. In addition, the ACS's 1950 film *Breast Self-Examination* was still circulating in 1972. It was screened for both secular and church women's groups, eventually being viewed by thirteen million women over the decades. Despite the startling fact that 95 percent of all breast lumps were first discovered by women themselves, BSE was still fairly unknown until Shirley's announcement.[41]

The boost BSE received as a result of Shirley's candor thrilled the ACS. A letter from the ACS president, Dr. Alva Letton, was among the thousands Shirley had received after her post-surgery press conference. In it, he wrote, "The American Cancer Society is deeply impressed and profoundly grateful for your forthrightness and honesty in emphasizing the importance of early detection of breast cancer."[42]

By 1974, because of the First and Second Ladies' surgeries, breast cancer again became a topical—rather than taboo—subject. Just as suddenly, BSE was discussed at length and everywhere: in newspapers and magazines, as well as on television. Some included a graphic showing the proper procedure; others featured actual (clothed) models. For the first time, women were empowered to take steps toward detecting such a feared disease. Like Shirley, they, too, could change their situation from passivity to activity.

Shirley's well-publicized story also inadvertently energized the second new breast cancer tool: mutual-help groups. Today we know them as support groups, but in 1972, they were a novel approach in the mental health world. As a species, humans are not solitary creatures; they share both good times and bad. People often find kinship in common suffering. It was on this premise that Alcoholics Anonymous—perhaps the most famous mutual-help group of all—was founded in 1935. Besides stressing anonymity, the organization is nonprofessional, unaffiliated, nondenominational, apolitical, and free to all.[43] It became the model many mutual help groups followed.

In the early 1970s, one could occasionally find "mastectomy groups"—an umbrella term for any organization whose theme was breast cancer, regardless of whether they focused on breast cancer detection and prevention or on recovery from mastectomy. Reach to Recovery was the first group to focus on the post-surgical period, founded in 1957 by Terese Lasser. With the attending surgeon's approval, volunteers met with women while they were still in the hospital. The volunteers had all had mastectomies themselves (and for decades, most of those were Halsted radicals), so they could speak from personal experience about the pure shock of having such a mutilating amputation.

The program also focused on exercises a woman could do (again, only with her physician's approval) to improve function in her arm and shoulder now that her chest muscles were gone. Reach to Recovery assistance typically ended a month or two after a woman returned home, leaving her to deal on her own with whatever other physical and psychological challenges she faced down the road.

A diagnosis of breast cancer (or any cancer, for that matter) is accompanied by a whirlwind of complex feelings. Many women felt left in a vacuum, forced to wrestle with their problems alone or, if they were lucky, with the help of a few family members. Mutual-help groups, on the other hand, became fellowships of survivors. Their woman-to-woman, shared experience led to the establishment of close personal bonds, enormously important both immediately post-surgery and for years to come. It was authentic interaction that couldn't be duplicated by the era's nearly all-male medical professionals. Furthermore, even after a woman became a "senior" member of such a group, in helping others she herself continued to heal.

⟿

By the time Rose returned from her research sojourn in Europe on December 15, she had already decided on the importance of including a chapter in her book on early detection. This was partially motivated by eye-opening comparisons she had discussed with every physician she met. If a woman in the United States went to her doctor after finding a lump, an all-too-frequent practice of general practitioners was to tell the woman, "Let's keep an eye on it." This widespread procrastination was eventually labeled "professional laxity."

On the other hand, in every country on Rose's aggressive three-and-a-half-week itinerary—England, Scotland, Sweden, Finland, and the Soviet Union—the doctors she met with told her that when a patient presented with a potential cancer symptom (lumps being the most frequent), they were immediately referred to an oncologist. There was no waiting.

The reason for the difference in approach between those countries and the United States was no mystery to Rose. Her nephew had recently passed his obstetrics-gynecology board exam. "His 'cram book,'" she huffed, "had two paragraphs about examining breasts."[44] No wonder doctors were so blasé; if textbook authors didn't think examining breasts was medically important, why would physicians? Rose would later write that while women might not be able to change the culture of professional laxity, they could certainly be proactive and make BSE as regular a part of their lives as washing their hair.

She had also decided her book would devote a chapter to the psychological healing that had to occur after breast cancer. In fact, Rose had outlined most of the book while traveling during her trip. The more she learned, the more she realized three things: how badly she had originally been treated; how truly well she had ultimately been treated; and that she would do everything in her power to ensure clear sailing for all women diagnosed with breast cancer in the future.

Chapter 7

~

Everyone Has a Story

On June 20, 1975, Americans met what would become the most famous shark in history. The production crew nicknamed him Bruce. To the public, he was known simply by his film's title: *Jaws*. Grossing $7,061,513 the first weekend (more than $41 million in today's money), the film completely overshadowed what might have otherwise been the biggest news that week.[1]

In January, the U.N. had declared 1975 as International Women's Year. To celebrate, the first-ever United Nations Conference on Women was held in Mexico City. The conference began the day before *Jaws* swam onto movie screens, opening with a welcome speech by U.N. secretary general Kurt Waldheim (secretaries general were always men). He was followed on the dais by the president of Mexico, Luis Echeverría Álvarez (in 1975, all but three heads of the world's governments were men). Echeverría then introduced the head of the host delegation, who, following U.N. meeting tradition, also always served as conference president. Consequently, at history's largest conference on women, after opening speeches by two men, it was presided over by a third man, Mexican attorney general Pedro Ojeda Paullada.[2]

Nonetheless, among the seven thousand delegates was the world's only woman astronaut, cosmonaut Valentina Tereshkova. She told reporters proudly, "The Soviet Union is the big exception in the world when it comes to opportunities for women, in politics, sports, economics and even space. The world would be better if men and women worked together."[3] If only.

Two thousand miles north of Mexico City, in Washington, D.C., a second June event would have an impact on American women. The proposed Title IX of the 1972 Education Amendments Act made clear that any education program or activity receiving federal funding must grant girls and women the same rights and opportunities as boys and men. However, the needle still hadn't moved. This amendment to the amendments, written in an urgent and nonnegotiable tone, was presented to Congress. Testimony from both those in favor of the revision and those against it was heard, and some of it became heated. While the focus of the testimony was primarily on how the changes would affect athletics across the educational spectrum, it further drove home the point that women could not, and should not, be excluded from any form of federally funded education, including medical schools. This was one more chapter in a very long story.

In his 1848 booklet *Man-Midwifery: Exposed and Corrected,* Dr. Samuel Gregory wrote, "The employment of men to attend women in childbirth . . . [is] unnecessary, unnatural, and injurious to the physical welfare of the community."[4] Dr. Gregory then went on to found the Boston Female Medical College. As America's first women's medical school, it opened with twelve students and two instructors. By this time, Dr. Elizabeth Blackwell was entering her last year at Geneva Medical College in New York. Having begun her education the year before Dr. Gregory's school opened, Dr. Blackwell would become the first woman to graduate from an American medical school. Her courage and drive in the all-male venue had been fueled by a dying friend who was convinced her care would have been better if it had come from a woman doctor.

At the dawn of the twentieth century, men's medical schools began admitting a limited number of women. But little standardization existed along the path to becoming a doctor. Some medical programs were attached to respected universities; others sprouted randomly, often lacking trained instructors. Consequently, the American Medical Association (AMA), then fifty years old, declared that a new century required substantial reform in medical education. It sought minimum requirements for graduation and longer training periods. The latter caused tuitions to rise, which in turn resulted in the evaporation of smaller institutions.

The AMA released a report in 1910 showing that women accounted for only 6 percent of all physicians in America. While the report clearly stated that "privileges must be granted to women . . . on the same terms as men," the increasingly stringent standards made access more difficult for women.[5] As a result, the number of female doctors remained unchanged over the course of the next fifty years.

When Rose's mastectomy was performed in 1974, there were 334,028 doctors in America. Of that number, only 25,401 (7.6 percent) were women.[6] Rose had seen for herself the accuracy of the Soviet cosmonaut's declaration about her country being the big exception in the world when it came to opportunities for women. She was further astonished to learn that there were more women doctors in Europe at the time than in the United States.

The Moscow stop on Rose's book research itinerary was the Institute of Experimental and Clinical Oncology. When she arrived in early December 1974, she was introduced to the head of the institute's all-female breast center staff, Dr. O. V. Sviatukhina (also a woman). The doctor was running a clinical trial on the efficacy of partial mastectomies (more than a lumpectomy but less than a simple mastectomy). These cutting-edge surgeries preserved more of a woman's breast, and while they were considered risky in the United States, in the USSR they were showing a survival rate similar to that of the all-encompassing radicals. Plus, chest preservation meant that surgery was a far less terrifying prospect to patients.[7]

Dr. Sviatukhina employed other procedures designed to improve her patients' post-cancer lives as well. She routinely utilized a procedure called a lymphangiography, injecting radioactive isotopes of gold into the lymphatic chambers between the fingers of breast cancer patients before their surgeries. The isotopes would only settle in healthy nodes throughout the body, skipping the cancerous ones. Thus, Dr. Sviatukhina was able to spare as many axillary nodes as possible, which would lessen ensuing lymphatic swelling of the arm.[8] (Today's sentinel node biopsy is usually performed during breast surgery and detects the first, or sentinel, lymph node, to be removed and examined to assess if cancer cells are present.) When Rose got to Leningrad, however, she found an all-male breast cancer team, staunch defenders of the Halsted mastectomy. They took all the axillary nodes—cancerous or not—without ever checking them in advance.[9]

Just as Dr. Blackwell's friend had felt that care from a woman doctor would have been better, Rose concluded that "having physicians who can empathize and sympathize because they, too, have breasts must be very supportive."

⁓

Jaws was still the nation's number-one movie when changing leaf colors and school buses signaled the arrival of fall in 1975. The women's sections of newspapers featured ads heralding Estée Lauder's autumn makeup colors, wedged among feminine-slanted news items. These sometimes included stories about the U.S. ambassador to Ghana, Shirley Temple Black, although her male colleagues were consistently featured in the front sections of the papers. More demeaning was that most articles still began with a reference to her childhood movie career, glossing over what she saw as her far more important diplomatic position. Ironically, within Ghana's Akan matrilineal society, women often played a larger role.

But while the media insisted on remembering Shirley's acting days, the impact of her breast cancer transparency still resonated with women. "Has Shirley Temple Black regained her health after having breast surgery for cancer a couple of years ago?" one asked in a syndicated write-in column. The answer delivered a mixed message. "Fully recovered, both mentally and physically, from the trauma of mastectomy," the unknown columnist responded. Following that high note, the writer continued that she was fully immersed in her role as ambassador. "And if the 'Good Ship Lollypop' still haunts the now-plump Mrs. Black, she says she doesn't mind at all: 'Because of my past, people think of me in a friendly context.'"[10] Snarky tone aside, the question illustrated humankind's persistent anxiety about cancer.

When Rose's book, *Breast Cancer: A Personal History and an Investigative Report*, arrived in bookstores three weeks later, it was precisely what the doctor ordered for that anxiety and more. While the cover was remarkably similar to the cover of Dr. Crile's book (the one that launched Rose's quest for more breast cancer knowledge), and that similarity might have been a deliberate tribute, the content was all Rose. It was comprehensive. It was understandable. The tone was a little indignant at times. Most importantly, however, it was the first book of its kind ever printed.

A journalist chimed that it was so expansive, it might have been titled *Everything You Wanted to Know About Breast Cancer, but Were Afraid to Ask.*[11] Dr. Dao wrote the foreword, marveling that Rose had begun this massive project just weeks after her own mastectomy. He, too, agreed that she was a pioneer. "As Mrs. Kushner knows, it is difficult to find a discussion on breast cancer for lay people that tells them all they need to know, and impossible to find one in which the disease . . . [is] adequately described and . . . which recounts one full human response to it from an actual patient's point of view. That is what Rose Kushner has done."[12]

Rose described her work more matter-of-factly: "What I did was translate the medical literature into plain English."[13]

That may have been her goal, but the effort to get there couldn't be overlooked. Aside from hours in the National Library of Medicine, Rose interviewed doctors and researchers at NIH, NCI, the U.S. Food and Drug Administration (FDA), the ACS, and more. Every time one of them mentioned another specialist, she hunted that person down for their thoughts. The research trip to Europe and the USSR gave her a different perspective. Countries whose medical and pharmaceutical regulations are less stringent (although no less responsible toward patients' health) allow for doctors to heal their patients with an eye toward quality of life. That point would become huge in the coming decade.

Following all that research was the massive task of organizing the material and then writing concisely, with an eye to the fragile state of a woman facing cancer. The book's first chapter, entitled "What Happened to Me," set the stage for all that was to come. Explanations of how cancer occurs, why it occurs, surgery types, and the healing process were followed by the lively chapter "Male Chauvinism, Sex, and Breast Cancer." The book's final chapters focus on the future, offering a beacon of hope for the eighty-eight thousand women who would be diagnosed in 1975, and for all those who would come after.[14]

Dr. Dao was among the many honored guests invited to the Kushner home the night after publication in 1975. The cocktail celebration was a cross section of friends and neighbors, doctors and researchers, and journalists. The party also gave Rose the opportunity to announce her next pioneering project: the Breast Cancer Advisory Center (BCAC).

The center was born at a lunch with her attorney in late 1974. She explained to him that since her *Washington Post* article had come out, she was being inundated with letters from women across the country asking for help. They had found lumps; what should they do? Their mother had had cancer; would they get it too? They had undergone mastectomies and felt ugly and isolated; whom could they talk to?[15]

Rose's heart broke for all of them. She knew their panic, which felt akin to being locked in a windowless closet with a known killer brandishing a weapon, the killer's hot breath on their necks. With nowhere to go, no weapon for defense, all they could do was hope for the best.

A call-in system, the Cancer Information Service (CIS), had been mandated by the 1971 National Cancer Act. It could have filled the void by educating the public, answering questions, and referring callers to the appropriate specialists and hospitals. But CIS wouldn't have been breast-cancer-specific; more to the point, it wasn't even operational. The only obvious solution, Rose explained to her lawyer, was for her to take matters into her own hands. *She* would be the information service. She asked for his help to set up what she thought would be a "temporary" nonprofit.

Nine months later, with Dr. Dao serving as chairman of the board, the BCAC was ready. Rose had a social worker and a clinical psychologist on hand, both of whom specialized in breast cancer issues. She had also hired Dorothy Johnston. As a registered nurse and the center's staff director, Dorothy answered the special phone they had set up in her home. (She gave her children orders never to touch it.) Piled high on a spindly little desk were ready references: books on cancer and lists of names and phone numbers of doctors who performed two-step procedures—and *didn't* perform Halsted radicals.

Beside those piles were the all-important fact sheets—photocopied pages from Rose's book on breast self-exam, diagnosis, the new mammography machines, and more. Like the book itself, it was information desperate women couldn't find anywhere else. All the services were free of charge, financed by donations and Rose's book sales.

Publisher Harcourt Brace Jovanovich had expected sales of Rose's book to be brisk, but their sales projections came nowhere near the fantastic reality. Accessible information on breast cancer from a survivor herself was to American women what water was to a parched traveler in a desert. Rose was packed off to more than sixteen cities, doing radio and television interviews, which were covered by the press. She appeared at bookstores to speak and sign copies. What had earlier been an inundation of letters became an absolute tsunami. And since it was an era where women's individual identities were usually given little importance, nearly all of the letter writers signed with "Mrs.," followed by their own first names in some cases, their husbands' in most cases.

A postcard (picturing an orange grove on the front) came from Venice, Florida, and read, "Dear Madam, I turned on your program late—didn't get the title of the book on cancer. Please send that to me." Mrs. Richard R. had signed the card.

Litchfield Park, Arizona, resident Mrs. Lee R. wrote, "I was impressed with your book and your talk on T.V. Would you please recommend a good chemotherapist-oncologist in Phoenix? Thank you."[16]

From Niagara Falls, New York, Mrs. Diane O. wrote, "Please send two copies of your book Breast Cancer. Enclosed is $10 for each and one dollar for their postage."

Mrs. Janie L. E. of Mine Hill, New Jersey, requested, "If you have any literature available concerning breast cancer, either free or at a small charge, I would very much like for you to send it to me. A self-addressed stamped envelope is enclosed for your convenience."

Despite the fact that many of the writers had heard or seen Rose in the media, and despite the fact that the organization was called the *Breast Cancer* Advisory Center, the convention of the time was to address inquiries to anonymous, faceless men. Some letters followed that convention. A Hartford, Connecticut, woman wrote, "Dear Sirs: Please send me all information on the best cancer treatment. Mrs. B.P.K."

Mrs. Richard L. from Houma, Louisiana, requested, "Gentlemen, Inasmuch as I meet all, or most, of the criteria for high risk category, I would appreciate any up to date information available on breast cancer and treatment." Covering the gender bases, Mrs. Karma M. of Huntsville, Alabama, wrote, "Dear People, What kind of information can you send me about breast cancer detection? Mechanical methods."

One of the sweetest messages came written on a circa 1975 IBM punch card from Mr. R.H.M.: "I would like to have further info on publications plus I would like to order the book that the woman was talking about on TV. I never heard her name or the book's name. Thank you. My wife would very much [like] to have this info."

Before long, the advisory center became a Kushner family project. Rose would bring home the mail from the center's post office box. Lesley (later accompanied by her friends) helped on weekends and during school breaks, going through the letters, sorting them into piles according to topic: questions, family history of breast cancer (Rose was interested in the possibility of a genetic link), requests for information, and so on. Donations came most often in the form of one-dollar bills, which Lesley would pile up for Harvey to count.

Before the center opened, and even after, women called Rose at home, no matter the time of day. It wasn't hard for them to track down her phone number, as in the directory she was listed as both Rose Kushner and Mrs. Harvey Kushner. In typical teenager fashion, Lesley was often first to the phone. When the caller would ask for Rose and start talking about her concern, Lesley would cover the mouthpiece and shout, "Mom! It's a lump!"[17]

Rose spoke to every caller and answered every letter. Without being the least bit aware, Rose had created a brand-new category of lobbyist: breast cancer advocate. She had also walked directly into the women's health movement, bringing breast cancer with her. After all, every woman in the movement had a pair that could, at any moment, go rogue.

⟿

The May 4, 1976, editions of American newspapers were filled with thousands of articles about the country's bicentennial celebration, exactly two months away. But there wasn't a single mention of the hearing about to convene in Room 4232 of the Dirksen Senate Office Building, across the street from the U.S. Capitol. That Tuesday morning, the Subcommittee on Health would begin hearing about the current state of affairs in breast cancer: what the best treatments were, where physicians differed, what risks and costs were involved.

Since 1971, the subcommittee had been chaired by Massachusetts senator Edward Kennedy. Early in his Senate career he had convened hearings about expediting research, which resulted in the 1971 National Cancer Act. Then, just two years later, Kennedy's twelve-year-old son and namesake was diagnosed with osteosarcoma in his right leg. To save young Kennedy's life, his leg was amputated above the knee.

Now Senator Kennedy was calling the subcommittee to order at 9:35. "The hearing this morning on the treatment of breast cancer is the first of a series of hearings that will occupy the Subcommittee on Health during the coming months," Kennedy told those assembled. "It is very appropriate that the first of these hearings be devoted to the treatment of breast cancer. This disease is one of the leading causes of death among women within the United States."[18]

The senator said they would hear about the necessity of radical mastectomies, one- and two-step surgeries, and the patient's right to share in the decision concerning the type of operation to have. "We hope that the expert witnesses . . . will not only help us to formulate more clearly these and other pertinent questions, but may help point the way to a solution to some of these important problems."[19]

The first "expert witness" welcomed was Rose. It was true: she was—unfortunately—an expert, and she knew the facts. She was comfortable delivering that information; by this time, she had been interviewed by dozens of print and electronic journalists. More remarkable was that she had acquired this status in less than two years, during some of which she was recovering from her own diagnosis and treatment.

Rose began her statement by explaining her cancer experience, admitting she was a rare exception. "Most women are not as lucky as I was. They have neither the background nor the advice I had, and they must blindly follow whatever procedure their physicians recommend."[20]

Addressing Kennedy's point about patients sharing in their treatment decisions, Rose pointed out, "In the United States, most of the 90,000 women who are expected to discover breast cancer in 1976 will be put to sleep without knowing whether they will wake up with one breast or two."

When the discussion turned to the efficacy of a modified versus Halsted mastectomy, Rose pointed out that modified mastectomies such as hers hadn't been done long enough to provide satisfactory data for some surgeons, who stubbornly insisted that survival rates needed study. Still, Rose told the senators, that didn't mean that just because a procedure had been done for eighty years it was better.

"From what I have read about Dr. William Stewart Halsted," she declared, "I am sure that if he were alive today, he would be the first person to put the mastectomy that bears his name on a museum shelf next to the leech." The use of the slimy, bloodsucking creatures to pull "tainted" blood from a patient had ceased about the same time Halsted began his radical surgeries.

Kennedy asked her if there was a difference in the insurance reimbursement to surgeons for the different types of mastectomies. Rose explained that she had done research into the California Relative Value Scale, a point system that had been devised by insurance companies to determine the price of a medical procedure. As Rose described it, each point had a different worth depending on where geographically the patient was seeking treatment. In Maryland, for example, a Halsted mastectomy was worth fifty-five points, while a modified radical mastectomy was worth only thirty. Rose maintained she didn't think surgeons made their decisions based on money. She figured they left the paperwork to others and often didn't even know what each operation was worth. Rather, she said, they were just going along with the status quo.

"I think they just don't know any better," Rose said, shrugging. "And I don't know if I'd rather have a greedy surgeon, or a dumb one."

The room erupted in laughter, the high note on which her first congressional experience finished. But she stayed until the end of the hearings. Next up was Dr. Frank Raucher, director of the NCI. He was accompanied by Dr. Bernard Fisher (who was still heading up the Breast Cancer Task Force) and Dr. Vincent DeVita, head of the Division of Cancer Treatment at the NCI. They, along with Dr. George Crile Jr., who followed them, spoke of the advantages of less invasive surgery, which in their opinion should then be followed by the new chemotherapy treatments.

Drilling to the heart of the matter, Kennedy asked Dr. Raucher, "If your wife had cancer of the breast, which would you advise her?"

The doctor never hesitated. "I would advise her to have a modified surgical procedure followed by chemotherapy."[21]

Cancer draws a line in the sand of life. There was the time before it, and all that comes after. Before her diagnosis, Rose's journalistic mantra was "Everything is a story." But after her cancer, and after the Breast Cancer Advisory Center began taking calls, she realized her real life mantra should be "Everyone has a story." And some of those stories were truly tragic.

A woman contacted Rose to say she couldn't bring herself to shop for new clothing because she feared that a saleswoman would see her mutilated body. Another married woman told Rose she was afraid that her mastectomy would drive her husband into the arms of a "whole" woman, since she was now just "part" woman. A man lamented to Rose that his wife had slashed her wrists as a result of being depressed after her surgery. Rose could see it did little good to tell these women that they had to lose breasts because their lives were at stake and they would have died otherwise. Some would have rather been dead.[22]

In the latter half of the 1970s, cancer was still seldom discussed publicly. And despite living in a mammary-oriented culture, where two—preferably large and shapely—breasts were thought essential for a woman's self-image, the psychological distress of losing those breasts was almost never brought to light. Some surgeons even thought it best not to tell a woman she had breast cancer, assuming her frail psyche would be unable to handle the news. Yet when surgery was over, those same doctors (and a great many more) couldn't understand why women were so distraught about their missing breast.

Rose freely admitted that the thought of cancer had frightened her. It had been, she said, "an automatic signal to order a cemetery plot and a tombstone."[23] But once she was past the shock of it all—and still at the Roswell Cancer Institute—she became overwhelmingly motivated to move past her own experience in an effort to help other women. Two decades later, Drs. Richard Tedeschi and Lawrence Calhoun would name the positive change that results from struggling with a major life crisis like cancer: post-traumatic growth. But in 1974, when Rose began interviewing women for her book, she realized that her state of mind was not the norm.

Of the 130 women Rose spoke with, the word most often used to describe how they felt during their treatment was "helpless."[24] Their testimonies led to her conceptualization of the four stages of emotional trauma from breast cancer. First was the moment the lump was found, its threat leaving the woman in unknown territory, with an unknown future. The second stage occurred when the doctor confirmed that something might be wrong and ordered nonsurgical tests (needle aspiration, mammogram, thermogram, etc.).[25]

The third stage, the wait between diagnosis and treatment, happened infrequently in 1974. After assessing the tests, some (unfortunately not many) doctors recommended only a biopsy to confirm cancer. If it was confirmed, waiting for the surgery in this two-step procedure was admittedly stressful. But those days or weeks before the mastectomy also gave a woman time to adjust psychologically to having cancer and to prepare for her recovery period after surgery. If a doctor offered only the one-step procedure, the fourth and greatest emotional trauma occurred: a woman would awake from surgery to learn that her breast had been amputated.

Doctors of the era were quick to tell their patients that, as with childbirth, where the memory of discomfort passes rather quickly once a baby is in its mother's arms, the more time that passed after a woman's mastectomy, the more the pain of losing a breast would recede.[26] Physicians routinely drew upon this time heals all wounds idea to dismiss the traumatic shock a woman suffered in a one-step surgery, when she awakened from a biopsy to find half of her chest wall gone. Their response was a pat on the hand and a solicitous "It won't seem so bad down the road."

Physicians could now also point to Betty Ford and Happy Rockefeller, who just weeks after their surgeries were photographed attending luncheons and celebrating holidays. The photos were always accompanied by quotes that they were "just fine," suggesting that if Betty and Happy could do it, so could anyone else.

While writing the chapter "After Surgery: Psychological," Rose couldn't help but consider her own mental state during and after her treatment. She hadn't wanted Harvey to see her scar right away. Ropey and red, its ugly puckering made her self-conscious. But then, after it had smoothed and lost its fiery hue, she shed her shyness. Undaunted, Harvey had steadfastly remained Rose's sounding board and most ardent supporter. That kind of love erased any feelings of unattractiveness she might have experienced.

And while she certainly hadn't sought the attention, an incident at her Moscow hotel during her research trip confirmed she was still attractive. An American businessman she had encountered in the lobby was persistent that she join him one evening. She declined his dinner invitation, but later she encountered him again in the elevator. He mentioned having been away from his wife for two and a half months, and when he discovered they were both on the seventeenth floor, he commented about the convenience of that fact. Rose had to suppress a laugh at the expression she imagined would have crossed his face if she had invited him in, whipped off her bra, and displayed the empty space where he expected a breast to be.[27]

Because of the large number of women she had spoken with, it was glaringly evident to Rose that her adjustment to cancer and surgery had been relatively smooth. Her research acumen, a brilliant and understanding doctor, and a loving husband had helped her make the best of a horrendous life event. Women without those resources had nowhere to turn.

Just as Rose had been putting the finishing touches on her manuscript in 1975, she read a report from the NCI stating that there were 677,000 women in America with a history of breast cancer. Her other research, however, based on material from Reach to Recovery and various newspaper articles, put the number somewhere between 300,000 and 350,000.[28] Where were those unaccounted-for women? And who were they?

Reach to Recovery's mission was to convince women that their mastectomies weren't permanent handicaps, as one representative described it to Rose. "We decided we would help the patient for just a few weeks, and then leave her to her own psychological recovery."[29]

The ACS, Reach to Recovery's parent organization, had long prided itself on educating the public about cancer. The same year as Rose's mastectomy, the society had enlisted Gallup to conduct a poll on women's attitudes toward breast cancer. Unsurprisingly, most of the 1,007 female respondents, all eighteen years and older, had never received any factual information about the disease and/or held gross misconceptions.

The survey also provided another significant (but, again, not surprising) finding. When asked if "breast loss can affect both a woman's self-image and her relationships with men," 61 percent of the single women surveyed and 66 percent of younger women (ages eighteen to thirty-four) said yes.[30] Yet the only treatment supported by the ACS's all-male breast cancer committee was the Halsted radical mastectomy.

In summation, then, the primary American organization charged with education about breast cancer discovered that women possessed either little factual information or misinformation about the disease. Those women strongly feared the eighty-year-old procedure behind which the organization insisted on rallying. And after having that procedure, they would be left to navigate any psychological issues on their own, which many did by hiding their surgery, or themselves. Clearly, those were the answers to Rose's questions of "where" and "who" with regard to the country's breast cancer statistics. She had just pulled back the curtain on the unacknowledged collateral damage of radical mastectomies.

⁓

"Public education is the domain of the American Cancer Society and all medical information is sieved through its filters before it is passed on. . . . We are told by the American Cancer Society only what the doctors want us to know."[31]

Firing these arrows directly at the ACS, Rose began her testimony before the House Subcommittee on Intergovernmental Relations and Human Resources. The June 14, 1977, hearing had been convened for an "in[-]depth review" of the National Cancer Act, which was now nearly six years old.[32] Rose explained to the congressmen that women were doing breast self-exams, as they had been directed. But when they found something suspicious and called either the NCI or the ACS, the standard response was always to call their doctor. She pointed out that general practitioners, along with their general surgeon counterparts, were busy with hernias, tonsils, and broken bones; they couldn't (or wouldn't) keep up to date on the advances in cancer treatment.

"The ACS is physician-oriented; it is not patient-oriented," Rose said. "As I stated earlier, the Society tells the American people only as much as physicians want us to know. Naturally, physicians do not want us to know more than they themselves know, and . . . they often don't know too much."[33]

Rose had attached thirteen Breast Cancer Advisory Center fact sheets to her written testimony, explaining her efforts to fill in where she felt the ACS was lacking. Her bigger point was that the American people were being short-changed. Taxpayers' dollars were supporting the NCI's research, but information about the results of that research—in this case, progress in the treatment of breast cancer—wasn't reaching those taxpayers.

"Why is the NCI so fearful of 'confronting' the ACS?" Rose asked. "I don't know. . . . The NCI was charged by the Congress with the obligation of keeping us Americans—NCI's employers—aware of everything our tax dollars have bought. If the ACS wants to help the NCI, this is fine. But the NCI must be the parent, *not* the obedient child."[34]

The combination of Rose's expertise and outspokenness was earning her a variety of labels. Her congressional testimony put her in the "expert witness" category. And when she was invited to speak at Baptist Memorial Hospital in Jacksonville, Florida, four months before appearing before the House of Representatives, journalists labeled her a "controversial cancer patient." The hospital was hosting a cancer seminar on February 2. Rose was hoping to teach the physicians and nurses in attendance that cancer looks very different from a patient's point of view. Because of an incident that occurred after the seminar, she would end up learning as much as she imparted.

At 3:30 the morning after the seminar, Rose was awakened from a dead sleep by an unfamiliar sound. It took a few moments for her to collect her thoughts. The bed she was on was in a hotel. The hotel was in Jacksonville. And the sound was the fire alarm. She jumped out of bed, switched on the light, and began putting on the clothing she had worn the night before, which included inserting her prosthetic breast into her bra. Then, grabbing a jacket, she carefully opened the door and stepped into the hallway, where she encountered other dazed hotel guests. They all made their way to the stairwell and descended to the lobby. In addition to the 240 guests of the hotel, the lobby was also filled with reporters who had been alerted to the blaze.

As Rose was helping herself to the freely flowing coffee, a reporter who had also been at the seminar the previous day recognized her. They chatted, and he stepped aside so a photographer could snap her photo. Then he asked her innocently, "I'd like to know why you bothered to get dressed when the emergency signal went off."[35] Rose looked around. Most of the nine-story hotel's evacuees were in some state of undress, wearing coats or robes over their pajamas. (She was pretty sure there was one man who was wearing his coat with nothing underneath.) The only people fully dressed were members of the media, the hotel staff, firefighters . . . and Rose.

Why *had* she gotten dressed? The answer was simple. Appearing "normal"—with two breasts—subconsciously took precedence, even in the face of a fire. Rose had thought she was without psychological scars. Evidently she was not.

Chapter 8

~

Freedom of Choice

"Closely matches the look, feel, and touch of natural breast tissue."[1] "Opening up your lifestyle and making you realize you don't have to be restricted because of breast surgery." "For women who've had breast surgery . . . answers."

In 1974 ads never mentioned the word *cancer,* and only rarely used the word *mastectomy.* But in shades ranging from pale ivory to rich cacao, with a nipple option or without, the array of breast prostheses was mind-boggling. All required a doctor's prescription. Even for a strong-willed woman like Rose, getting up the nerve to begin the search hadn't been easy. After she had waited the customary six weeks for her incision to heal, it took her three weeks to begin shopping.

The silicone-filled plastic forms she was offered looked and felt like human flesh, and were certainly an upgrade from what had existed in earlier decades. In the 1950s, women were able to move past bras stuffed with cotton batting, bags of birdseed, or balled-up nylon stockings when the Dunlop Tire Company produced rubber breasts. They looked reasonable, but they were hard and caused the wearer to sweat. The 1960s saw American ingenuity introduce inflatable breasts, but manufacturers hadn't considered the downsides. The balloons were prone to deflating suddenly, sometimes with a great deal of noise—causing women to carry straws in their purses for emergency reinflation. Airline travelers had the opposite problem. The drop in cabin pressure as the plane ascended caused the air inside the prosthesis to expand, sometimes explosively.

In the early 1970s, a Bavarian plastics engineer began experimenting with new materials to form a more natural and modern version of a breast prosthesis. His successful creation drastically changed the lives of millions of women.[2] However, the new kinds of prosthesis often weren't available in the lingerie sections of department stores; when they were, most saleswomen were untrained in both the product and the customer, and as a result were often unable to conceal their shock when they saw a mastectomy site.

A second option was to visit surgical supply stores, where the pseudo-breasts sat wedged between wheelchairs and crutches. Female clerks were a rarity in those stores, so already traumatized women customers had to work with male prosthetic fitters. As the aforementioned ads suggest, mail order options existed, too, but they left much to be desired when it came to accurate color and size.

It was fortuitous, then, that at the same time prostheses were being refined, so were techniques for sculpting the breast. Plastic surgery was born out of the necessity to repair facial wounds suffered in the battles of World War I. Even if wounded veterans were physically capable of working after their recovery, a hole where a nose or cheek had once been affected their employability. The ability to do surgical repairs turned those whom society had once considered "monsters" back into humans. That concept was stretched for patients (primarily women) whose facial features, or the ravages of age, made them unattractive by conventional standards. Sales pitches proclaimed that the beauty achieved by plastic surgery created well-being, and thus healed the patients of their presumed inferiority complexes.

And then came an even greater stretch. If women's breasts could be made more beautiful, think of the possibilities! That was precisely the quest of Texas doctors Frank Gerow and Thomas Cronin, the pioneers of silicone breast enlargement. Their work during the 1960s changed lives. Some of the newly enhanced women were actresses, models, or exotic dancers. But others were just ordinary wives and mothers who no longer wanted to be flat-chested. And while artificial breasts were certainly not appreciated by the bra-burning women's movement, breast-obsessed men around the world were eminently grateful.

Up until that era, reconstructing breasts after mastectomies had not enjoyed much success. Various surgical attempts included using a patient's own fatty tissue, taken from the hips; or making a mound of the pectoral muscles (if the muscles hadn't been cut away); or bisecting the opposite breast, giving a woman two half breasts. The new silicone implants seemed like a logical, and brilliant, solution. However, most plastic surgeons were male. And just like many other doctors of the time, they couldn't relate to the psychological damage of losing a breast. Consequently, they couldn't relate to the restoration of one, either.

Some doctors thought breast reconstruction was a frivolous surgery. Others became downright indignant. When an Indianapolis woman asked her doctor about reconstruction, he exclaimed, "My God, woman, how vain are you? I just saved your life!"[3] Major insurance companies (also a male-dominated industry) refused to cover the cost of such "vanity" operations. They would soon learn what a mistake that was.

In quiet Rapid City, South Dakota, Patricia Koppmann existed in a depressed cloud after her mastectomy.[4] Then one Sunday in 1976, she read a story about a Des Moines, Iowa, surgeon who was performing reconstructive surgery. Patricia contacted him, and after a consultation, he told her he felt very good about her case. Surgery was scheduled for November. But when Patricia made a claim to Blue Cross and Blue Shield of Western Iowa and South Dakota for her $12,000 surgery ($66,500 today), they denied coverage for what they called a "cosmetic" procedure. So in August 1979, the thirty-seven-year-old launched what became a landmark case in discrimination. Five months later, the insurance company agreed to cover all of her surgery and legal costs.

But that wasn't all. "I had made up my mind I would not just settle for the money," Patricia said. "I wanted a . . . policy change."[5] On January 27, 1980, all of the nation's 115 Blue Cross and Blue Shield plans agreed to cover the surgery. With Patricia's case in the books, other women filed suit against their insurance companies, too.

A greater benefit was waiting in the wings. If women saw that they might be made whole again, perhaps fewer would be afraid to report suspicious lumps to their doctors. Only a few hundred American women had had reconstruction during the first half of the 1970s. But by the time Rose had hers in early June 1978, the procedure was becoming more popular and accepted, with twenty thousand survivors receiving new breasts by 1981. Rose maintained, however, like all decisions regarding breast cancer, reconstruction was a very personal decision.

Aside from Rose becoming cognizant of her appearance insecurity after the Jacksonville fire, the final straw for her reconstruction decision had occurred in a bargain department store. She bent over to pick something up off the floor of the mass dressing room, and her prosthesis fell out. "Look mommy," yelled a little girl, "that lady's booby fell down." Rose was mortified.[6]

Of course she had done her homework prior to surgery. Her implant was a sealed pouch of sterile saline. The news surrounding silicone implants of any kind wasn't good on a number of fronts, including that the silicone "migrated" to other parts of the body. When Rose perceived that big companies, like Dow Chemical, were recommending their silicone for reconstruction implants, her antennae went up. Distrusting their motives, she explained simply, "No one's making money on salt water."[7]

～

When *Breast Cancer* had come out in 1975, Rose was certain that her chapter on the dangers of the Pill and the need for patient cancer warnings would cause a congressional firestorm. Instead, its effect was akin to an extinguished match: no fire, no storm, and no change in package inserts. In her ongoing effort to whip up interest, she also contacted the FDA, offering to testify should the agency convene hearings. She was given time to speak, but it fell on deaf ears and nothing changed. Now that the executive branch of government had failed, her next step was to contact the legislative branch. Despite having a Maryland senator as an ally, she found that there was still no appetite in Congress to pursue her cause.

Harvey joked about her approaching the remaining branch of government, the judicial.[8] She didn't see it as a joke and began contacting women lawyers to see if any might take the case pro bono. While none of them said no outright, they all said "not now," because they were swamped with other work. Even the ever-growing collection of feminist organizations were a dead end, citing the necessity of having the membership vote before pursuing any legal endeavor—something that Rose figured would be time-consuming and fruitless.

And then providence intervened. Martin Baron, a New York personal injury lawyer, called. He had read Rose's book and hoped she could help him with a malpractice case he was working on. She agreed, and then, never a shrinking violet, asked for his help. After she'd laid out what she was hoping for, he barked, without any hesitation, "When can you get up here?"

"I've got no money to pay you," Rose told him.

"So who asked you for money?" he shot back, laughing. "This is more important than any of my other cases. Let me know when you'll be getting in and I'll pick you up."[9]

Baron had his work cut out for him. First he had to find precedents proving that a private citizen could sue an executive agency, which the FDA was. He found them. Next, since Rose lived in Maryland and he practiced law in New York, he had to find a co-plaintiff living within his licensure area. He found that, too. Prominent New Yorker Marlene Manes was a friend who had once been a Pill user. She was happy to join the case. Baron also found a Commerce Department regulation stating that if a prescription drug listed one adverse side effect—manufacturers had given in to adding the warning about blood clots among some Pill users—it had to list *all* the potential side effects. And that would include the increasing evidence about breast cancer.

On September 26, 1976, their suit was filed against FDA commissioner Alexander Schmidt and Health, Education, and Welfare (HEW) secretary F. David Matthews. New York Eastern District Court judge Thomas Platt would preside. In her affidavit, Rose maintained that if the Pill really wasn't dangerous, why not say on the bottle that it had not shown an increase in breast cancer? The government countered, claiming it was a bothersome overkill, requiring new patient literature to be printed. The legal wrangling went on so long that the defendants had to change as Ford's presidency became Carter's.

While Baron was neck deep in the legalese, Rose was hardly idle. She solicited quotes from doctors who agreed with her. She traipsed around Baltimore with prescriptions for oral contraceptives (each for a different brand) to learn exactly what literature was being dispensed. And she rounded up crucial witnesses: women who had been diagnosed with cancer after having been on the Pill. Some spoke anonymously, some allowed Rose to use their names, and some died before seeing justice done.

When Judge Platt wrote his final decision on February 3, 1978, it was in Rose's favor. The new patient packaging would read: "Women who have or have had . . . cancer of the breast or sex organs should not use oral contraceptives. . . . The estrogen in oral contraceptives has been known to cause breast cancer and other cancers in certain animals. These findings suggest that oral contraceptives may also cause cancer in humans."

Rose had hoped the warning would also mention that the Pill would be dangerous to women with a family history of breast cancer. But as she acknowledged in a letter to Judge Platt, "I accept the wording of the patient labels as published, because they are too vital to postpone." In the same letter, she spoke from the heart. "On behalf of all women, I would like to thank Your Honor for your great role in expediting the publication of this final ruling."[10]

Rose calculated that Baron's costs must have come to at least $10,000 (in excess of $48,000 today). But he never charged her a dime. As a memento, she gave him a Lucite paperweight with a month's supply of oral contraceptives embedded in it, and a framed copy of the new patient package insert. If she had been keeping score, it would have read Rose Kushner 1, medical establishment 0.

~

When Rose walked into the NIH's Masur Auditorium at 8:30 a.m. on June 5, 1979, she wasn't the least surprised to see that she was the only woman. Nor was she concerned to see that she was the only non-physician. She had known those things in advance. She was determined, however, to be more than just the token patient at this Consensus Development Conference.

The NIH had begun convening these meetings two years earlier. The intent was to bring together medical professionals and researchers in an effort to reach general agreement on the safety and efficacy of medical technologies, which included surgical procedures. This particular meeting—the seventeenth of its kind—was to answer the question "Are there clinical alternatives to the radical mastectomy that minimize patient morbidity and yet do not decrease a patient's survival potential?" Their decisions would drive breast cancer treatment protocols in the future.

Because Rose had often done research at the National Library of Medicine, she had become a familiar face to others on the NIH campus, including then–deputy director Dr. Seymour Perry. He had called Rose earlier in the year to invite her to join the June panel She was flabbergasted. Less than five years earlier, she had been seen as a lunatic for bucking the Halstead practice. She couldn't help but ask Dr. Perry if he was joking.

"Of course not," he said. "This will be a chance for you to say what you've been saying for more than four years. But this time, you'll be talking from a National Institutes of Health stage. If you're too scared to do it, I'm sure I can get someone else."[11] Now she was embarrassed, and she eagerly agreed to participate.

All panelists were asked to submit a summary of their formal position on the question at hand. Rose sent hers (discussing her disdain for Halsteds) to Dr. Perry, sending a copy to Dr. Dao at the same time. He called her two days later, fuming: "You have no business talking about whether or not a woman needs a certain kind of operation." While he acknowledged she knew a great deal about breast cancer, she had never been, he stressed vehemently, standing over a patient with a scalpel in her hand.

Rose was taken aback by his anger, telling him that she hadn't written anything that she hadn't already said dozens of times before. "And Dr. Perry asked me to be on the panel specifically to give a patient's point of view," she explained.[12]

He restated his position on her speaking about medical matters, but by that time he had calmed down. It made no sense, he pointed out, to just reiterate what the doctors would say. "But there is one way for you to make a real contribution that will probably not even be thought of by anyone else on the panel," he offered. "You must write a new summary to replace the one I have just read. But in this one, you—as a patient—should urge that there be a separation between the diagnostic biopsy and whatever definitive treatment the surgeon might decide is necessary."[13]

He was right, of course. And for whatever reason—postal efficiency or something more mystical—her presentation summary had arrived in Dr. Dao's Buffalo, New York, mailbox before it had been delivered to the NIH, five minutes away from her home. When she drove over to Dr. Perry's office to retrieve her original document, the envelope hadn't even been opened. She wrote a new summary and shipped it off.

The meeting's official title was "The Treatment of Primary Breast Cancer: Management of Local Disease." Its panel was a diverse assemblage of doctors, some of whom Rose knew and some she didn't. Along with representatives from across the United States, France, and Italy were Dr. Jerome Urban, Happy Rockefeller's surgeon, and Dr. Bernard Fisher, whom Rose had interrupted at the September 1974 breast conference held in the same auditorium. In the five years since, she had peppered him with questions and phone calls, and a mutual respect had grown. Dr. John Moxley III, a pediatric oncologist from the University of California, was the coolheaded moderator of this "science court," which would soon become very heated.

Each panelist laid out his case for or against the ninety-year-old surgical dinosaur. Half of the American women diagnosed with breast cancer that year would undergo Dr. Halstead's aggressively mutilating procedure. Dr. Fisher and others in favor of a modified mastectomy vociferously argued that cancer was now much better understood than in Halstead's time. The premise that cancer grew progressively outward, in the same way an apple rots, had been replaced with the knowledge that the deadly cells travel via blood and lymph fluid. The doctors also provided data showing that the newer surgery's survival rate was the same, and in some cases better. By contrast, there was no data to support Halstead's notion of "getting it all out" by hacking away more.

The group finally came to a consensus (although one doctor claimed to have been railroaded) and produced their statement: "The Halsted radical mastectomy should no longer be the treatment of choice for local breast cancer. . . . The new standard of treatment is to be the simple (or total) mastectomy in which the breast is removed, a sampling of the underarm nodes is taken and the pectoral muscles are left alone."[14]

At this point, the men in the room had done what they came to do; they might have tried to ignore the only woman, and the only non-MD, among them. They were in for a surprise as Rose began her presentation. Over the past year, she said, the government had rolled out a campaign encouraging patients to seek a second opinion before deciding on surgery. President Jimmy Carter had proposed that Medicare and Medicaid require and pay for such a step. Even the American Medical Association had advocated for this "heretical" idea in an effort to cut down on malpractice suits. Second opinions were becoming the norm for every type of surgery but one: the mastectomy.

"Usually, when the decision is made to perform a mastectomy, the person most concerned is unconscious," Rose said, explaining that the woman would first have been told by her surgeon that whatever her breast abnormality, it would have to be cut out. "She probably signed some papers giving the surgeon permission to do whatever he thinks is necessary should cancer be found." That "whatever," of course, included removing her breast. If such haste meant saving a life, there would be no argument. But experts knew that by the time something could be felt in the breast, it had been growing for at least two years. A few more days or weeks would make no difference.[15]

"No man is going to make another impotent while he's asleep without his permission," Rose pointed out, "but there's no hesitation if it's a woman's breast."[16]

More time between biopsy and surgery would allow for more analysis of the tissue. If the cancer had spread to other parts of the body, a mastectomy would be unnecessary. More time would give doctors an opportunity to ascertain if a woman had underlying conditions that needed to be considered before such major surgery. More time might even allow the woman's own immune system to attack the cancer and shrink the tumor. Most important, more time between biopsy and surgery would give a woman the opportunity for a second opinion.

Rose read the room and could tell she was gaining some ground. Pressing her advantage, she reiterated the point that studies were showing that survival and recurrence rates associated with two-step surgery were virtually identical with the rates associated with one-step surgery.

The debate continued for hours, but Rose would not be dissuaded. The long, difficult, and not always congenial discussion was in some aspects not unlike the jury deliberations portrayed in the iconic 1957 film *Twelve Angry Men*. Just as Henry Fonda's character was the only person on that fictitious jury who believed in the innocence of the defendant, Rose's had been the only voice on the panel to point out that "no woman should be wheeled out of an operating room with one breast when she had expected to have two."[17]

It was an idea most (male) doctors had never considered. Gradually, as had happened in the film, with the other jurors coming around to Fonda's point of view, the other participants in the panel conceded Rose's argument and ultimately wrote a second, unexpected consensus statement: "There should be a time lapse between the biopsy of suspicious breast tissue and any 'definitive surgical procedure' to treat the newly discovered breast cancer."[18]

The 107,000 women who would face down cancer in the next twelve months, along with all those who would come after, had just been given the freedom to choose the course of their own healthcare.[19] In fact, states would begin passing informed-consent laws, ensuring that patients received information about all possible treatment options. The score now was Rose Kushner 2, medical establishment 0.

⁓

In 1961, the movie studio 20th Century Fox had a problem. After a string of box office flops, the company was short on cash. But it had a great deal of real estate in downtown Los Angeles. So it sold 180 acres to a developer, who created Century City, with the Century Plaza Hotel rising in its midst nineteen stories high. When the hotel opened on June 1, 1966, every one of its 750 rooms offered cutting-edge luxury, including air-conditioning and a color television set. With a presidential suite offering views all the way to the Pacific Ocean, the Century Plaza was marketed as the "world's most beautiful hotel." Nearly five years to the day of its opening, however, it would also earn a spot in breast cancer history.

The National Conference on Breast Cancer convened its second meeting at the hotel on May 17, 1971. For three days, the host, the American Cancer Society, provided 1,300 doctors an opportunity to mix, mingle, and hear from experts on their shared goals: to prevent, treat, and cure breast cancer. Topics ranged from possible viruses and the Pill's contribution to the disease to the remarkable results of an eight-year clinical trial on breast imaging.

Mammography was still a relatively new and developing weapon in the anti-cancer arsenal. Its heritage began in 1896, when German physicist Wilhelm Roentegen discovered X-rays. Over the ensuring decades, some experimenting was done in imaging the breast with X-rays. But it wasn't until 1960 that MD Anderson doctor Robert Egan made a huge breakthrough. Refining the intensity and quantity of radiation used, plus experimenting with different types of film, Dr. Egan was able to reliably produce high-quality mammograms. (Machines created specifically for breasts didn't appear in the United States until 1967. Consequently, early mammograms were performed between X-rays for broken legs and strained backs.)

The stage was set for Dr. Philip Strax, whose first wife had died of breast cancer in 1947 at the age of thirty-nine. In 1962, Dr. Strax had approached a prepaid medical plan, the Health Insurance Plan (HIP), with his idea of a large, long-term study to test the efficacy of mammography. Happily, the NCI was interested in the same thing, and funded Dr. Strax's work. Sixty-two thousand women between the ages of forty and sixty-four were divided into two groups. One group would receive the standard physical breast examination, and the other group would also receive a mammogram.[20]

The findings that Dr. Strax and his team would now present at the National Conference on Breast Cancer were astonishing. Not only did the group receiving mammography see 40 percent fewer deaths from breast cancer, but 70 percent of those who were discovered to have breast cancer were diagnosed before the disease had spread to their lymph nodes. Plus, 33 percent of the breast cancers had been found by mammography alone.[21]

Following the Century City Hotel meeting, Dr. Strax approached the ACS with a bold plan, ultimately called the Breast Cancer Detection Determination Project (BCDDP). Hundreds of thousands of women nationwide (ranging in age from thirty-five to seventy-four) would receive free annual screenings, including a physical examination, mammography, thermography, and instruction in self-exams. The ACS board formally endorsed the BCDDP in February 1972, and the whole thing was paid for by the NCI at a cost of $10 million a year ($75 million today). Since the heady gold rush established by the National Cancer Act had just begun, this seemed a good use for "Nixon's Christmas gift to the nation," signed just two months before. Because of the flood of calls in some areas from women intent on saving themselves from their most feared disease, some women had to be put on six-week waiting lists to receive their screenings.[22]

Gradually, however, concerns were voiced. What medical issues might the radiation used in mammograms cause down the road? A "safe" level hadn't yet been determined. Long-term effects from the atomic bombs dropped on Japan less than thirty years earlier, however, did show that radiation caused problems, breast cancer among them.[23] And who was reading the films once they'd been taken? There was no standard for radiologist training in mammography yet in existence. Lastly, was there really a need to screen women under fifty? Despite the fact that breast cancer was the leading cancer killer of American women, and the leading cause of death in women aged thirty-nine to forty-four, breast tissue is typically denser in younger women and therefore more difficult to see through without higher doses of radiation.

The person with the loudest voice on all of this was one of NCI's own. Dr. John Bailar III, an epidemiologist and editor of the *Journal of the National Cancer Institute*, had gone on a one-man speaking tour across the country, publishing a number of serious critiques of the program. "[There is] a possibility," Dr. Bailar said, fanning the fires of concern, "that the routine use of mammography in screening asymptomatic women may eventually take almost as many lives as it saves."[24]

BCDDP had other problems, too. Even though mammography machines were now being produced by a number of American manufacturers, there were no standards regulating how much radiation the machines should emit. For example, Ralph Nader's watchdog organization, the Health Research Group, discovered that the machine at Georgetown University Health Center was emitting three times the "safe" level, per their own private research. But that was just one opinion. There wasn't any standardized training for the technicians operating the machines, either.[25]

Both the NCI and the ACS publicized information about mammography, but much of it was conflicting. This caused the exasperated NCI director, Dr. Frank Rauscher, to call together the institute's three hundred women employees to ask their opinion about mammograms. After the hour-long discussion, 45.6 percent of them felt they would be willing to have a mammogram, while 31.7 percent said they wouldn't. The rest were undecided. Ironically, this was the first time a group of women had been asked their opinions about breast imaging—anywhere, ever.[26]

The discussion would be a long one. It was, in fact, this very controversy that caused NIH to convene its first Consensus Development Conference in September 1977—the same conference where Rose would make history two years later. The final statement from the inaugural meeting was that mammograms should be done on women between thirty-five and thirty-nine only if they had a personal—not family—history of breast cancer.[27]

The controversy would not end there, however. Nor would Rose's participation in it. (How was it that she had become a medical controversy magnet?) But referring to Dr. Bailar, years after his Paul Revere–like 1976 alarm regarding mammography, she was clear: "Women all over the world are indebted to him for disobeying one of the cardinal rules of bureaucracy: 'Don't mess around in anyone else's turf.' Because of him," Rose continued, "low-dose x-ray film was perfected, more special-purpose mammography equipment using film-screen was acquired by radiologists, and more care is taken by everyone involved."[28]

⟶

By 1980, Rose had garnered many titles. From the unwelcome mantle of "breast cancer patient," she had more or less stumbled into "breast cancer advocate." Her writing—always a combination of memoir, how-to handbook, and manifesto—earned her the "expert witness" title at congressional hearings. Rose's story had evolved into a living demonstration of advocacy. Consequently, tackling all of these battles on the breast cancer front brought her a new title on March 25: that of member of the National Cancer Advisory Board.

As mentioned earlier, the NCAB had been created by the 1971 National Cancer Act and was something near and dear to Mary Lasker's heart. Her most ardent initial desire in helping to stimulate cancer research was that the NCI be removed from NIH and stand on its own like NASA, reporting directly to the president. While the first part of that proposal ultimately wasn't accepted, NCI was given the distinct advantage among its sister institutes of direct presidential communication. Mary's second desire was an advisory board that would oversee all things related to American cancer research. That board—whose members would be appointed by the president—would prepare an annual report for the president.

Mary stood fast on her belief that the NCAB had to include representatives from the general public who, "by virtue of their training, experience, and background, are especially qualified to appraise the programs of the Institute."[29] That was certainly Rose, who gratefully accepted the appointment from President Jimmy Carter. And she was in great company. Among the other non-scientist appointees that year who would serve a six-year term was Mary's good friend Eppie Lederer, otherwise known as Ann Landers.

Of course, Rose also held the title of founder of the Breast Cancer Advisory Center. She had recently received a $30,000 seed money grant from a small Washington, D.C., foundation. In addition to offsetting the cost of sending out her fact sheets, Rose was hoping to print more copies of her information booklet, *If You've Thought About Breast Cancer.*[30] The NCI had been buying large quantities of the booklet—they had even asked for a Spanish translation—and in turn made certain it was circulated to cancer centers, doctors' offices, and other logical locations. Rose also sold the pamphlet to banks, insurance companies, Bell Telephone, and General Motors for their female employees.

The biggest dream she was able to realize with the seed money was being able to move the whole operation out of her house and into a commercial building. She found a four-room suite of offices on Rockville Pike just four miles from her home. Harvey secured unused desks and file cabinets from his company. And the Raytheon Corporation donated a Lexitron word processor, which allowed updates to the fact sheets to be made much more easily—no longer did she have to completely retype entire pages every time information changed or something new was discovered.

BCAC's new offices had a counseling room where a social worker could speak with walk-ins (free of charge), and a receptionist to greet them. Dorothy Johnston could also now work away from home, with an office to handle incoming calls. Plus, there were desks for the volunteers who handled myriad tasks.

On move-in day, Rose and one of the volunteers, Mattie (who was also a breast cancer survivor), flirted brazenly with the building's very handsome manager, batting their eyelashes and giggling like teenagers at his jokes. Their efforts scored extra parking spaces for Mattie and Dorothy. The women laughed afterward: "Do you think anyone would belive this? Two women with missing breasts trying to flirt parking spaces out of a man!"[31]

Everything was flowing so smoothly. Vital breast cancer detection, treatment, and survivorship information was getting into the hands of American women. The NCI's purchases of the brochures were funding subsequent printings. The BCAC was operating like a professional organization. And then, like rising water in a flood, governmental bureaucracy seeped in.

Ronald Reagan had focused a good deal of his 1980 presidential campaign on the American economy. He promised to make drastic cuts in what he called "big government," which would in turn allow him to deliver a balanced budget to the American people. After his landslide victory, he began working toward those promises, and his budget for fiscal year 1982 (which began in October 1981) included cuts in printing. Because the NCI is a part of the government, they were impacted by these cuts, and they obeyed the law by canceling their order for 100,000 copies of *If You've Thought About Breast Cancer,* which would have been delivered in January 1982.

The cut was bad enough, but the knowledge that not all government agencies were playing by the rules enraged Rose. She was quite sure that the Departments of Agriculture and Defense were still getting money to cover printing costs. Even the National Heart, Lung, and Blood Institute had found a publication work-around. (Heart attack and lung cancer were the leading killers of men.) Frustratingly, the NCI appeared to be the only agency that was really adhering to Reagan's print moratorium. As the cash stopped flowing, the BCAC was forced to make tough decisions.[32]

⌒

The "thing" on Rose's chest had begun like an ordinary pimple. Red at first, tender, and then developing a whitehead, it was, as she described, "four inches southwest of my Adam's apple." It wasn't on the incision of her removed breast, but near it. She put an antibiotic cream on it, got a prescription for an oral antibiotic from her doctor (who assured her it was nothing), and waited for it to disappear. It didn't.[33]

Rose was in the middle of a press tour promoting the new and updated version of her book. She had also changed the title from *Breast Cancer* to *Why Me?* in order to overcome public denial about the disease—reporters had told her they put other covers on the original version in order to read it on the subway, and women who bought it asked bookstores to bag it and then bring the bag to the cash register to ring them up. She complained, "While women are ready to read about vaginal deodorants, soft bowel movements and rape, we aren't ready for a book boldly titled *Breast Cancer.*"[34]

After taping a television interview on May 25, 1982, Rose was in her plastic surgeon's mini operating room on June 10 to have the "thing" removed. He promised to get her the biopsy result the next day so she wouldn't have to worry over the weekend. However, the pathology report didn't come in until the following Monday, when the doctor called her.

"I'm sorry, Rose," the doctor said softly. "Something must have kicked up a dormant cell."[35] The cancer was back. That "something" might have been the stress under which Rose put herself, marching forward in her breast cancer crusade, slaying dragons at every turn. She was bucking a powerful medical establishment, taking on speaking engagements coast to coast, and writing furiously, now less for mass media and more for scientific journals. "I would love to write for the magazines women read," she explained, "because that's a good way to get to women."[36] But those magazines always wanted her stories to end on a happy note, and sometimes stories didn't.

In fact, that was the most difficult part of all for Rose: listening to the stories of women whose lives weren't happy, women who never returned to normal, women whose husbands left them, women who died of their disease. When it became overwhelming, Rose sometimes dissolved into tears.[37] But then Harvey would intervene in his loving way, and she would emerge to fight again. Still, she paid a price for her relentless advocacy. Just eight years and one day after finding her original lump, Rose was again diagnosed with cancer.

She was scared: did this mean the disease was metastatic, the second-most-frightening word after *cancer?* She was angry: everyone knew that five years cancer-free meant you were out of the woods, you were cured. She was dogged: as before—but this time, much more knowledgeable and with a huge list of cancer luminaries as allies—she went on a quest for information.

Every doctor she saw (including Dr. Dao in Buffalo) told her chemotherapy, in the form of one of the new drug cocktails, was probably the way to go. And the person to speak with was Dr. Marc Lippman, then head of NCI's Medical Breast Cancer Section, who possessed an enormous amount of chemotherapy research experience. Lippman was a straight shooter in the best of cases, but when Rose caught up with him, he was also rushing to catch a plane.

"Look Rose," he told her gently. "You are now . . . metastatic."[38]

That word. That horrible, terrifying word. It was the first time anyone had said it to her. And it meant that for the rest of her life, no matter how long that was, she would have cancer. "I reached behind me for a chair, so I would not fall from shock," she later wrote. Then, returning to a phrase she had once used with regard to her first diagnosis, she continued, metastatic "patients have to reserve cemetery plots and headstones."

Dr. Lippman explained the type of combination chemotherapy he would use with her and said he would begin immediately. "That's hitting a mosquito with a Sherman tank," she joked feebly. "What's left if this concoction doesn't work?" Dr. Lippman told her there were other effective compounds that they could try next.

"What about the studies showing that drugs change DNA [in some cancer cells] and start a drug-resistant strain that no other drug can kill?" Rose asked. Dr. Lippman told her that data was preliminary.[39]

The doctor caught his plane, and the patient buried herself in chemotherapy research. It appeared that the cancer-killing, albeit toxic, chemicals were also mired in controversy. Then she read about another option, tamoxifen, that could halt the growth of breast cancer cells that needed estrogen to grow. Created in 1962 by the Imperial Chemical Company, it had originally been thought to be a potential "morning after" pill. But in the 1970s, the estrogen modulator was found to have the opposite effect: it *increased* fertility. By 1978, however, its effectiveness in treating metastatic, estrogen-receptive breast cancer, as Rose's was, had been proven. (Dr. Elwood Jensen had first made the discovery that some breast cancers possessed estrogen receptors in 1973. That research had begun to be universally accepted when Rose began fighting for cancer warnings in birth control pill literature.[40]) Plus, tamoxifen had been shown to have fewer side effects. Now, four years later, tamoxifen was the workhorse for stage IV patients.

Rose believed that benefit always had to be weighed against risk. In the end, she decided to gamble. "That's what all breast cancer patients must do today," she wrote.[41] She would take only tamoxifen and hope that one pill a day would keep the cancer away.

Chapter 9

~

The Most Beautiful Discoveries

Five weeks and three days after Rose was officially diagnosed with metastatic breast cancer, Nancy Brinker was hosting a dozen women at her lovely home in suburban Dallas. They were "smart, capable, and fabulous," and willing to venture out into July temperatures that tickled one hundred degrees. Each had come because breast cancer was personal to them. It was the first official gathering of what would become the Susan G. Komen Breast Cancer Foundation.[1]

The story actually began five years earlier. Nancy's sister, Suzy Komen (three years her elder), had found a lump in her breast. It was different from the others that she had had; unlike them, it wasn't just a cyst. The doctor who had just done a needle biopsy told her he needed to remove the whole thing to determine exactly what it was. By the time Nancy could get from Dallas to her hometown, Peoria, Illinois, the mysterious lump had been diagnosed as cancer.

Suzy was content to have her surgery done locally. The doctor performed a subcutaneous mastectomy, which in essence was a deep incision, through which he scooped out the cancerous tissue, leaving the outside of her breast intact. After surgery, the very self-assured doctor announced to Suzy's husband, Nancy, and their parents that he had worked his magic and, after an implant to be inserted ten days later, she would be turned back over to society as good as new, with no need for further treatment.

Only Suzy wasn't as good as new. For six months, Nancy had encouraged her to seek a second opinion. And then Suzy found a lump under her arm. She agreed to go a large cancer research facility, where further scans showed that in addition to a metastasis to the lymph nodes, cancer was also in her right lung and elsewhere. Suzy had thirty rounds of radiation, which only seemed to further ignite the cancer's growth.

As a Texas resident, Nancy begged Suzy to visit MD Anderson Cancer Center in Houston to see if the doctors there had something new they could try. It was only when a physician friend suggested the same thing to Suzy that she went. As the weeks of treatment became months, the two sisters were disheartened by the dreary waiting rooms, with their old magazines. Suzy kept saying that "when she got better" they'd work on fixing things up. Over time, Nancy realized that Suzy was really saying "after I'm gone." She made Nancy promise to work on helping other women diagnosed with cancer, and to improve the journey for them and their families.[2]

Suzy died on August 4, 1980. She was thirty-six, a wife, and a mother of two.

Like Rose, Nancy became a woman on a mission, living her life in three parts: as a single mother, earning a living, and entrenching herself in cancer-related charities. After she married Norman Brinker—the brilliant mind behind restaurant chains Steak and Ale, Bennigan's, and Chili's—Nancy had a true partner in her quest to fulfill her promise to Suzy. Norman told her that people don't care about causes, they care about people.[3] That was the easy part. Suzy's would be the face of the organization. But its focus was still fuzzy.

In addition, an adage her mother had coined repeated itself in Nancy's mind: "Go where people aren't; do what's not being done."[4] Research was important, of course. However, breast cancer was still a disease only whispered about. It needed the light of day. It needed advocacy and support services. Nancy had no idea where to begin, and sought advice from Suzy's oncologist at MD Anderson, Dr. George Blumenschein, who had become a good friend. He encouraged her to go to cancer seminars, so she did.

Having determined that her foundation should be built like a business, Nancy thought partnering with a large, well-defined organization seemed a logical next step. She attended the Baylor University Hospital breast cancer symposium in the spring of 1982, and at the first coffee break she sought out the American Cancer Society senior officer who was in attendance. After listening for a few minutes, he told her that ACS would be proud to take whatever money she might raise, but they couldn't take on a breast-cancer-specific project. If they did, every other cancer would want one, too. Avoiding more attention to the leading cancer killer of women in America seemed a poor excuse to Nancy.

Retelling that story to the women who met for tea in Nancy's home that July afternoon further ignited their drive to do something, anything, about breast cancer. They decided their first fundraiser would be a fall lawn party at the Willow Bend Polo and Hunt Club.

Nancy later wrote, "Of course, speaking the very words 'lawn party' is probably the most effective rain dance ever devised."[5] Sure enough, the day of their big event, she awoke to a dark, wet, gloomy morning. No one would put on their best garden party garb and venture out on such day. Nancy grew even more heartsick when she arrived at the polo club. All the lovely pink decorations—she thought the feminine color was the perfect signature hue for a disease that affected mostly women—they had put up the day before were beaten down by the rain. They looked like Nancy felt: defeated. She had let her sister down.

And then, on the horizon, she saw them. A steady stream of vehicles turned onto the drive and wound their way up to the clubhouse. Hundreds would assemble that day, in memory or honor of someone, or just because they knew no woman on earth was immune to breast cancer. Collectively, they gave birth to America's first national breast cancer organization.

⁓

"The most beautiful discoveries are made not so much by men as by the period." These words are said to have come from the prolific German writer Johann Wolfgang von Goethe. The precise source aside, they couldn't be more apropos in a discussion about breast cancer. They certainly applied to Halsted's mastectomy. And they applied to the hornets' nest Rose poked in 1984 when she weighed in on the relatively new chemical darling of cancer treatment.

The birth of chemotherapy had occurred decades earlier. In 1943, at the height of World War II, a German bombing run over the harbor in Bari, Italy, sank a dozen ships. Worse, one of them was secretly carrying lethal mustard gas, which spilled into the water. The blistering wounds of the floundering survivors and their rescuers intrigued Dr. Stewart Francis Alexander, who was already researching nitrogen mustard (a relative of mustard gas). In addition to burning skin, nitrogen mustard also depleted white blood cells in research mice. (White blood cells are a bodily defense against infection.) When Dr. Alexander examined the sailors exposed to mustard gas, their white blood cell counts were also low, mimicking those of the mice. Perhaps, he postulated, a lesser amount of the gas could kill the cells of childhood leukemia (a blood cancer), without leaving the patient defenseless. His theory proved to be correct. Thus, from that deadly chemical weapon of war, the first chemotherapy agent—methotrexate—was created. Its successful use against childhood leukemia led to more experimentation and an expansion of usage.[6]

While the drugs did, indeed, kill the rapidly growing cancer cells, they also attacked other rapidly growing cells—namely, those in the stomach, the mouth, and the hair follicles. While a large dose of these chemicals slowed or halted cancer's spread, the nausea, mouth sores, and hair loss were difficult for patients to tolerate. The challenge for researchers, then, was to ascertain how much was too much.

Doctors who administered chemotherapy were known as "chemotherapists" until 1972, when oncology officially became a subspecialty of internal medicine. Their "angels in white" were variously called cancer nurses or chemotherapy nurses until 1975, when the Oncology Nursing Society was born. Meanwhile, new research showed that combining drugs became an even more powerful tool. Chemo cocktails were Dr. Marc Lippman's specialty and had been his offering to Rose at the time of her recurrence.[7]

Rose had written about the success of chemotherapy in the late seventies, when it was being used in only 7 percent of breast cancer cases. By the eighties, the usage had jumped to 22 percent.[8] This pro-chemotherapy movement caused Rose to change her views. Reading journals and attending oncology conferences, she was puzzled by (and cautious about) chemo's automatic and indiscriminate use. Aside from the well-documented side effects, studies were questioning chemotherapy's effectiveness in postmenopausal women, whose cancers were thought at the time to be less aggressive. There were darker potential side effects, too. New primary cancers occurred in some patients, and, as she had brought up to Dr. Lippman, there was the terrifying suspicion that the drugs might create a mutant strain of cells resistant to everything currently in the anti-cancer arsenal.

As sometimes happens in relationships, Rose's previously contentious one with the ultra-conservative American Cancer Society had evolved. This was not an unusual phenomenon for her. She was never shy about pressing her stance on issues, sometimes being harsh and even demeaning. But she would customarily follow those gunfights with a letter written in her characteristic self-deprecating and humorous tone. Since she had written just such a letter to the ACS, she wasn't surprised when Dr. Arthur Holleb, editor of their magazine, *CA: A Journal for Clinicians*, approached her asking for an "anti-article" on the subject of chemotherapy. Rose began writing furiously.

The draft of the article she submitted, "Is Aggressive Adjuvant Chemotherapy the Halsted Radical of the '80s?," initially began with an anecdote (which was later removed before the article was published): "'My patients never vomit,' a smiling oncologist told me at a recent conference. 'I don't know why, they just don't.'" In the article, Rose continued sarcastically, "I almost asked him if his magic also prevented baldness but decided to be quiet." And the attack was on.

Most of the country's doctors, she wrote, spend little time with non-life-threatening patient problems, and most oncologists don't even see their patients during routine appointments.[9] Rose pointed to a 1983 study in which doctors and their breast cancer patients were asked to complete identical twenty-question surveys. There was agreement between doctors and patients on only four of the questions, and vast discrepancies on questions that measured treatment toxicity, physical and psychological adjustment, and social activity.

Calling it the "red-badge-of-courage syndrome," she continued in her acerbic tone, "Glue a stylish wig on your pate, chew some Rolaids, and grin and bear it. Never hint to the doctor that the breast cancer medicine is the reason you feel sick."[10] Chemotherapy had become so routine—and in some cases was so extreme—that it wasn't a stretch for Rose to draw a connection between its usage and doctors' Halsted habit. Furthermore, this was happening with alarming speed. "It took almost a century to abandon the Halsted radical, but fewer than five years to embrace adjuvant [additional or auxiliary] chemotherapy."[11]

The big question was why. Rose blamed the results of an Italian study that she thought had been published prematurely. But she was equally certain that doctors were sometimes overeager in their work. "I object to the fact they dream up protocols over the urinal, and then go out and try them on people," she wrote to a friend a month before the article was published.[12]

While Rose was comfortable in her writing style, this journal was a different and uncharted ocean, and her words were not well-received. Some doctors wrote her directly, citing her article as "unethical" and "sheer egomania."[13] But two took their objections back to the very journal that had published Rose's article in the first place. In a response written to the editor of the journal, Dr. Lippman and his longtime research partner, Dr. Bruce Chabner, declared that "a number of issues she [Rose Kushner] raised require rebuttal."[14] Rose had apparently not considered that oncologists might be offended, particularly Dr. Lippman, whom she knew well.

They challenged her statement about chemo's benefit with studies and statistics, and did the same with her statements about potential drug resistance. They produced other evidence about the selection of patients receiving chemotherapy. But in their last argument, Rose saw that she had hit a nerve. "Ms. Kushner has implied a cavalier indifference on the part of the American medical community. . . . We believe that this is an unacceptable and global characterization of a group of physicians who have voluntarily chosen to provide for the needs of some of the most difficult . . . aspects of human disease."[15]

Rose might have been well served by a modicum of restraint in her attack on the profession. Most of those in the field were truly motivated to unravel the mystery that was cancer. Whether they envisioned becoming the hero who would cure it or simply wished to relieve a patient's suffering, their mutual goal was to save lives.

The entire saga, however, had beneficial and far-lasting benefits. Every time Rose encouraged patients (particularly women, who tended to be more reticent in their doctor's presence) to question *everything*, she was further expanding the patient-as-consumer model she had pioneered. Her courage gave breath to a new generation of breast cancer patients. And while she had written that *she* preferred to eschew chemotherapy and take only tamoxifen, she remained consistent in her belief that every decision about breast cancer and its treatment should be the patient's own.

Again the score changed: Rose Kushner 3, medical establishment 0.

⌐

Phil Donahue, who was once described as a combination of circus giant P. T. Barnum and hard-hitting journalist Edward R. Murrow, had begun his career in 1957 as a radio production assistant in his hometown, Cleveland, Ohio. The next step was to a morning anchor spot at a Dayton television station, and then, in 1970, his own daily program, *The Phil Donahue Show*, which he eventually moved to Chicago.

After a decade in the Windy City—where he earned more than a dozen Emmys, a Peabody Award, and syndication in two hundred markets—Donahue packed up his show and headed to the Big Apple. He was so popular, the waiting time to become an audience member in New York City was seven weeks. Which meant that when his Wednesday, March 18, 1985, program began, audience members were thrilled to finally settle into their seats.

Over the course of his career, Donahue had interviewed the now-missing Teamster boss Jimmy Hoffa, John F. Kennedy when he was a candidate for president, and civil rights activist Malcom X. But on this day, he was taking on an unlikely duo.

Rose and Dr. Marc Lippman hadn't seen each other face-to-face since her article had appeared in *CA*. She wasn't aware of his rebuttal, which wouldn't be published for another two months. But there they were, sitting just two feet apart, on Donahue's stage, ready to speak on a topic for which they were both eminently qualified.

Donahue prepped the audience with breast cancer's alarming facts and statistics. After introducing a somber Dr. Lippman, he turned to a smiling Rose. "And of all people, a woman is here to talk about this issue. Rose Kushner has seen this movie."[16] He asked her about her particular treatment, which she explained.

Donahue, the "hard-hitting journalist," followed her explanation by saying he was frustrated that medicine was so slow to change. In her congressional testimony nine years earlier, Rose had said she didn't think physicians made surgical choices based on what they might earn. Time had caused her to reverse that stand. Consequently, she had a ready answer: "Insurance companies could help if they paid differently. The Halsted might have been abandoned many, many years before if they had simply said, 'Look, you wanna do a modified or a Halsted, fine, but you're gonna get paid for the modified.' The Halsted earned more money for the surgeons." A collective intake of breath could be heard throughout the audience. It was the kind of reaction Donahue, "the circus giant," lived for.

He spun around and, microphone in hand, trotted over to a young woman seated near the front. "I think it's really great that women are questioning the medical community," she stated confidently, "and they're not just accepting what a doctor is telling them. There's information available, and that's really good." Dr. Lippman agreed that Donahue's program was important, and Rose added, "Information is therapeutic," affirming her belief that the more a woman understood about breast cancer in advance, the less traumatic it would be if she was diagnosed.

Running to the other side of the studio audience, Donahue took a comment from a woman about lumpectomies. They'd been done for years in Europe, the woman reported. Rose explained that she had discovered that, too, ten years earlier when doing research for her book. And as it happened, she said, an NCI press release had just been issued two days earlier, reporting on a ten-year comparison study of women with early breast cancer. The results showed that the rate of recurrence (or lack thereof) was the same across the three groups studied: total mastectomy, segmental mastectomy (the medical community's name for lumpectomy, a word reporters had coined years earlier), and segmental mastectomy with radiation.

Dr. Lippman chimed in about his own similar study on lumpectomies. The sincerity in his face supported his words. "I am very committed to trying to develop the safest, the least radical, the least mutilating surgery possible." What woman wouldn't sign up for something that erased her cancer and left her chest landscape intact? Clearly Dr. Lippman was on their side.

When a question about mammography came up, Donahue turned to the doctor, asking about radiation levels. The doctor responded, "I think the new data suggests that mammography is safe."

"You *think?* You *think!*" Donahue, the "hard-hitting journalist," asked incredulously, eliciting an eye roll from Dr. Lippman. Rose came to his defense. "Benefit has to outweigh risk. You can't worry about leukemia developing in twenty years if you have cancer now."

Donahue wouldn't back down, citing the emotional toll women were experiencing around breast cancer, given the advice they were hearing about how to be vigilant in advance and then the advice about what to do if they found a lump.

"Having breast cancer is no piece of cake," Rose interrupted him. "What can I tell you—it's tough!"

Dialing back the drama level, Donahue asked her whether she agreed that at least the nightmare of the one-step procedure was over. "Unfortunately not," she replied. It had been seven years since Rose's words had persuaded the NIH panel to proclaim the two-step procedure as a best practice. "Last year, according to the American College of Surgeons, more than 50 percent of the breast surgeries in this country were one-stagers." This time, the audience's responses were audible gasps.

Weaving through the rows with his microphone, Donahue stopped at a woman who asked, "What is even the legitimacy of a woman undergoing a biopsy and waking up finding that her breast has been removed? Why would that even happen?"

Like a moth to a flame, Rose couldn't resist her pat answer. "The doctor won't lose the business. She can't go to another surgeon."

Having heard about what *doctors* were telling their patients, about insurance companies paying *doctors* more for a Halsted, about *doctors* not losing money, one woman in the audience had had enough.

"I resent that!" she yelled. Attractive, well coiffed, impeccably dressed, accessorized with gold earrings and bracelets, the camera had picked her up earlier in a number of shots. Now "the circus giant" scurried up to the fifth row from the back, where she was sitting, and held the mic in front of her.

"My husband is a physician. You may know doctors who perform that way, but I know decent men who wouldn't do that to women."

Rose shook her head and said it was done every day, but the woman pushed on. "Well, as in every profession, I am sure there are some who don't live up to the Hippocratic oath. But the doctors I know don't operate that way. Their primary concern is to heal, and they do it the best they know how." Dr. Lippman spotted an ally in the woman, and he interjected that he, too, didn't agree with characterizing the entire medical profession as jerks. It was perhaps the perfect outlet for his frustration over Rose's article, and he was rewarded with applause. Rose's poise and smile never faded.

After twenty-five minutes, Donahue announced the first commercial break, saying, "We are in New York City with Dr. Marc Lippman and Ruth Kushner, and we'll be right back." Rose's eyes shot toward him. How could he have gotten her first name wrong? She opened her mouth to correct him, but it was too late. Messages from Ogilvie home perms, Grape-Nuts cereal, and Mrs. Smith's pies awaited. When the cameras again rolled, Donahue joked to ease the previous tension. "Do you know the most-often-performed unnecessary surgery in the U.S.? Circumcision!" Genuine laughter followed from the audience. He was so good at his job.

The last bone of contention came in the form of a discussion about radiation therapy. A woman in the audience related her tragic story of treatment with a lumpectomy and radiation that had gone badly, causing serious aftereffects. As had also been the case in the early years of reading mammographies, standardized training for radiation therapists was also slow to materialize. Assuming lack of training had been at play in the woman's case, Rose explained, "There are about two thousand board-certified radiation therapists in the country, but only two hundred have had experience [with radiation after lumpectomy], as they've never had the opportunity to do it on an intact breast."

"I hate to stir up controversy for no end," Dr. Lippman jumped in, "but I really don't agree with that." He nodded toward Rose; now it was her turn to roll her eyes. But after he finished his point that there were plenty of trained radiologists, he turned to the woman and said, "I am truly sorry that you've had a bad result. You said there was nothing that could be done. I don't believe that's ever true. Please call me."

The woman was flabbergasted. "No one has ever told me they were sorry. Thank you." That one moment spoke volumes about Dr. Lippman. His level of knowledge combined with his level of empathy was a rare combination in his field. Rose saw it, too.

—

Although the targets of Rose's wrath often were men, she wasn't aiming at them *because* they were men.[17] No, Rose's target was the medical community. It was just an unfortunate coincidence that the majority of them happened to be men. And when it came to illness, whether as physician or as patient, men's and women's responses to the same situation were often quite different, as in so many other aspects of society.

A male doctor and his female patient (wearing a surgical gown) were the focus of a medical school lecture in 1963. She had undergone a radical mastectomy in 1948 and the two were now sitting next to each other on the lecture hall stage. After the doctor finished his summary of the surgery, a student raised his hand. "What was the psychological effect of the surgery? Did the patient have feelings about losing her breast?"

The question was answered by the surgeon, who explained that the extensive operation was the woman's only chance against her breast cancer. As he spoke, he opened the woman's surgical gown completely, revealing a cavernous scar on one side of her chest and an intact breast on the other. Lifting the latter in his hand as if it was an object of curiosity, he assured his audience that the cancerous breast had "no cosmetic value." The woman, invisible to her healer as a feeling human being, never spoke or moved.[18]

This is, again, evidence of physicians being products of the period in which they lived. But it is no less heartbreaking. Much of the problem had commenced in medical schools, where women were routinely regarded as a subgroup of humans, unseen and relegated to an epidemic of neglect. Within textbooks and classrooms, there was little actual training on their bodies, although women would likely represent half of the new doctors' patients. Male physiology was the standard upon which all diseases and treatments were studied. That mindset was then carried forth when students became doctors, and it didn't stop with the body. The psyche was also dragged into the mire.

A female medical student commented in 1974, "Women's illnesses are assumed psychosomatic until proven otherwise."[19] As the country marched toward the promising twenty-first century, many doctors' opinions of women's health remained in past centuries. The reality was often that a woman's emotional issues were more likely to be the *result* rather than the *cause* of medical issues, not the other way around.

A frequent complaint from doctors was that they were "tired of neurotic women with nothing wrong with them who come in because they are lonely or dissatisfied with life."[20] Yet tragic examples disprove this sentiment. In 1987, three women independently went to three different emergency rooms complaining of breathlessness and panic symptoms. All three were diagnosed with hysterical hyperventilation. Two were referred to psychiatrists and one was simply sent home. Three days later, they returned to those same emergency rooms in various states of consciousness. Upon further examination, all three had untreated diabetes.[21]

Around the same time, another woman began a new job, which, in her words, "was difficult." After several months in which she was anxious, tired, and experiencing severe abdominal cramping, her physician, a man, diagnosed irritable bowel syndrome. She returned to the doctor a number of times, and each time the symptoms were routinely written off as the stress of her job. When the woman finally sought an opinion from a woman doctor, testing revealed that the patient had colon cancer.

Many women had believed their doctors who had said the lumps in their breasts were only something to be "watched." And when a surgical biopsy was finally scheduled, the last thing those women heard from their doctors before being anesthetized was that the lumps were likely nothing and everything was fine. Yet tens of thousands awoke missing one or both breasts.

So prevalent had this practice become that in 1988, American psychologist Brendan Maher coined it the "Martha Mitchell effect."[22] Martha was the wife of U.S. attorney general John Mitchell, fallen President Nixon's right-hand man. She insisted to the press that the White House was using her husband as a scapegoat during the Watergate scandal. In addition, she claimed she had been drugged and held against her will in a California hotel to keep her from speaking out. All of her accusations were written off as the ranting of a madwoman. But after her 1975 death from multiple myeloma, it was proven that Martha had told the truth.[23]

Rose had surely experienced the Martha Mitchell effect when she discovered her first lump and her doctor told her it was nothing to worry about. To be sure, she would have been just as angry about his demeanor regardless of his gender. Decades later, women's health concerns would still be written off, resulting in misdiagnosed heart disease, cancers, and other life-threatening issues. The practice may have new monikers, including "psychologization" and "gaslighting." But the result is the same.

"The first time I met Rose was at a breast cancer symposium in San Antonio," Nancy Brinker recalled. "I was standing among some scientists, and Rose marched right up, all 5 feet 2 inches of her. And the first thing she said to me was something about [me] being a socialite. It shocked me out of my wits, and it also offended me."[24]

Rose took no prisoners when it came to advocacy. She knew about the Susan G. Komen Breast Cancer Foundation. And she knew about Nancy Brinker, seeing her as one part breast cancer advocate, one part wife of a wealthy man, and one part friend to important people. Rose thought Nancy had the makings of a powerful ally—but only if her passion was genuine.

Nancy continued, "And then I realized what Rose was saying to me was, if you're really interested in this cause, if you really want to do something, you'll join the fight, and you'll use whatever resources you have to fight it with me."[25]

They met again while testifying at a congressional hearing in October 1985, and it wasn't long before they became good friends. Rose was one of Nancy's staunchest supporters, dismissing detractors by saying, "People are jealous because she's rich and beautiful."[26] It made sense that Nancy's name came to Rose as she mulled over the idea of bringing together breast cancer organizations under a single umbrella. She knew that together, they could have much greater influence.

In April 1986, the two women and a handful of others founded the National Association of Breast Cancer Organizations (NABCO). Their hope was to become a resource for anyone with concerns about the disease, as well as to have an impact on public and private policy, and on health legislation. Over the course of the next several years, Nancy and Rose became more than advocates; they were co-combatants trying to gain ground against a most mysterious and pernicious foe.

⟶

"What are we going to do?" The excited, raspy voice at the other end of the line had a drowsy Dr. Bernard Fisher confused. It was seven-thirty on the morning of October 16, 1987.[27]

"About what?" he asked.

"Mrs. Reagan has breast cancer and they're going to take off her breast. We have to make sure she knows her options."

Rose, after being notified by friends in the White House, was on the phone from the time she hung up with Dr. Fisher until 11:30 p.m. She called everyone she knew who might be able to get through to the Reagans or the doctors. All to no avail. It was September 1974 all over again. A First Lady was marching off to

Bethesda Naval Hospital to have her breast amputated. Mrs. Reagan had told her surgeons not to wake her up if the tumor proved to be cancerous. Just get it over with, she instructed.[28]

It took surgeons fifty minutes to remove Mrs. Reagan's tumor—about the size of a peppercorn—and the rest of her breast. After the president had visited, he told reporters that she was "resting comfortably" and feeling "the normal discomfort after an operation, but nothing more than that." Easy for him to say. He had never seen the two feet of his colon that had been removed two years earlier because of a cancerous polyp. His wife, however, would stare at her half-empty chest for the rest of her life.

Mrs. Reagan's doctors were pleased with her recovery, saying no further treatment would be necessary. But other breast cancer experts said the quick removal of her breast was "old-fashioned and unnecessary." They felt her modified radical mastectomy was a "most aggressive form of treatment for such an early stage of malignancy." Dr. William Goodson proclaimed, "It's a decision we might have made in 1957, but not in 1987 . . . and doesn't necessarily present a good example for women having to make such a decision."[29]

Rose, of course, was even more direct. She worried about women bothering to even get a mammogram to catch early and small tumors. The woman who could have the best treatment in the free world had just undergone the same procedure for a peppercorn-sized tumor as she would have had if it had been the size of a lemon.

She was also shocked at the rush to perform a one-step procedure. Without a doubt, Rose told reporters, the First Lady has "set us back ten years." She continued, "I don't want women to feel the president's wife got the best. The president's wife got what the president's wife wanted."[30] Mrs. Reagan got to make the call. That was, at least, one battle won.

⤙

"It's the dirtiest business in the world," Helena Rubinstein famously said of the beauty industry.[31] She was right. Competing brands waged constant wars, employing everything from head-on battles to sneaky guerrilla attacks. And in the center ring were Leonard and Evelyn Lauder. When Estée Lauder was a small company, it was easy to respond quickly to market trends. As Leonard later said, "We were more agile . . . and the big guys didn't notice until it was too late."[32] Company sales had soared from $50 million in the 1970s to $700 million in 1980.[33] And their most challenging foe yet arose: Lancôme.

The company had been founded in France in 1935, first selling perfume and then expanding into skincare. When the founder was ready to sell, Estée Lauder was interested, but the French didn't want their illustrious brand leaving the country. So the French mass marketer L'Oréal (then a $7 billion company) was happy to embrace Lancôme, which they then dropped on America's doorstep in 1981. The Lancôme wars were on.[34]

Whatever Estée Lauder did, Lancôme copied, from two-page spreads in glossy magazines to television prime time. Estée's pioneering gifts-with-purchase promotions could be had at Lancôme counters, too. Estée Lauder had pioneered using a glamorous model as the face of the company; Karen Graham had occupied the position since 1970. Lancôme also jumped on that bandwagon in 1982 with Isabella Rossellini, daughter of actress Ingrid Bergman. These were trying days for the Lauders.

Still, Evelyn remained the consummate juggler, managing her career and motherhood with grace. She had always been present for her sons, making it a point to be home by four o'clock every day when they were little. Now that they were grown men, she still relished an opportunity to be a support for them. It was no surprise, then, that in the fall of 1988, she had rearranged her calendar for a trip to California. Gary, twenty-six, was entering Stanford Business School, and she wanted to be on hand to help him settle into his apartment.[35]

Among the appointments Evelyn had needed to reschedule was her annual mammogram. At fifty-two, she was as diligent about them as she was about her skin care. Having returned home from California, getting the scan back on her calendar was no easy task in the midst of the Lancôme wars. And it still hadn't been rescheduled in November when she found the lump in her left breast. As it is for all women, it would be the moment that would completely redirect her life.

The pathology report after Evelyn's lumpectomy showed that her cancer was stage II (cancer is staged from I to IV, depending on the size of a tumor and how far the cancer has spread).[36] The next step in her treatment would be overseen by the hospital's well-regarded oncologist. The conventional chemotherapy he recommended was to begin on Monday, a few days after her Thursday surgery. Leonard was shocked by Evelyn's resignation to simply accept the path laid before her, without further investigation.

This was the woman who had fled Nazi occupation and lived through a terrifying race against time out of Europe. She was the woman who had remained at a party surrounded by Leonard's old girlfriends because Estée had asked her to, and then brought her sense of courage and dogged determination into the family business. Most of all, Evelyn was the love of his life. He couldn't possibly allow this experience to progress without knowing that she was getting the best treatment from the best person possible. And he needed time to find that person.

Fate's intervention in life is mysterious and unexpected. Evelyn developed an infection at the surgical site, which, in turn, caused her chemotherapy to be put off for one week. That was the window Leonard was hoping for; he had seven days to find the best. Among those he telephoned in his search was Dr. Ezra Greenspan, an oncologist friend at Mt. Sinai Hospital in New York. Dr. Greenspan was highly thought of, a brilliant doctor who was, in fact, treating his own wife for breast cancer. However, he told Leonard that if he had it to do again, he would have sent her to Dr. Larry Norton, who was about to leave Mt. Sinai for Memorial Sloan Kettering Cancer Center.[37]

The moment the short, bespectacled man in a white coat flew into his Wednesday meeting with Leonard and began to explain what he thought Evelyn's course of treatment should be, Leonard knew he had found the right person. Dr. Norton was as passionate about his cutting-edge cancer research as he was compassionate about his patients. But when Leonard returned home to share his excitement with Evelyn, she assured him the plan already in place was the way she wanted to go.

Leonard said that the cancer wasn't just *her* disease. They were a team, and thus it involved them both. They talked from lunchtime until two the following morning when—either because of fatigue or just to shut Leonard up or both—Evelyn finally agreed to see Dr. Norton. She later said she never realized how deeply Leonard loved her until that moment in their lives.

Chapter 10

~

And Now We Cannot Be Quiet

Greenwich Village was a mecca of music in the 1960s. And for Larry Norton, it was just a cheap subway ride from home. He had a great ear and a talent for multiple instruments, but he was particularly drawn to the electric guitar. After high school, Norton headed upstate to the University of Rochester, a "hotbed of musical inventiveness," as he would later call it. But with a little more maturity, Norton realized music might not be the most lucrative career, and he began looking for an alternative.

A friend had just completed an "inspirational" summer internship with Dr. William Regelson, an early pioneer in chemotherapy at Roswell Park Memorial Hospital. (In 1972, two years before Rose became a patient of Dr. Dao's there, it was renamed Roswell Park Cancer Center). The word *inspirational* caught Norton's attention, and he headed to Buffalo to interview with Dr. Regelson. Norton's description of his experience was that it was "eye-opening." More specifically, it was career-launching.[1]

After graduating from Rochester, Norton earned his medical degree at Columbia University, trained in internal medicine at Albert Einstein College of Medicine in the Bronx, and then became a fellow at the National Cancer Institute. While at NCI, he became curious about cancer recurrences. Researching tumor growth, he came across the Gompertz equation (a mathematical model that describes the growth of an entity or movement as being slowest at the beginning and end of a given time period), developed by British mathematician Benjamin Gompertz early in the nineteenth century. Applying the equation to the vast store of animal data at his disposal, Dr. Norton discovered that smaller cancer tumors actually grew faster than larger ones.

Then, in 1979, together with his colleague Dr. Richard Simon, he developed what came to be known as the Norton-Simon hypothesis, which posits that cancer cells are killed by treatment at a rate that's directly proportional to the rate at which they are growing at the time of that treatment. The corollary is that the most effective treatment plans are "dose-dense." In other words, the two doctors believed that giving patients chemotherapy doses as frequently as could be tolerated, and sometimes sequentially rather than simultaneously, would have better results than the then-current protocols.

Dr. Vince DeVita, director of the NCI at the time, explained with classic precision how the Norton-Simon hypothesis affects chemotherapy protocols: "We give chemotherapy on days one and eight, and we give radiotherapy five days out of seven. Why? Because that's the schedule that conforms to a five-day work week. But tumors are smarter than that. We need to think about what's driving the growth of the tumor. And if that means giving the treatment at 2 a.m., then that's what we have to do."[2] Cancer, as he pointed out, doesn't take weekends off, and neither should the doctors.

Although the Norton-Simon hypothesis was at first considered blasphemy, it would come to be known as the greatest innovation in cancer treatment in twenty years. And it was this difficult and riskier—but more promising—treatment that Evelyn agreed to undergo with Dr. Norton at MSKCC.

The most accurate way to describe the day the doctor and patient first met in late December 1988 is with a cliché: the stars aligned. Evelyn immediately saw Dr. Norton's passion for making sure she wasn't one of the forty-five thousand women who would die of breast cancer in 1989. And she could relate to his passion; it was a twin to hers, which had propelled her forward in the beauty industry. Their mutual zest for life fueled a bond. Or, as Dr. Norton later said, "We had a deep and immediate friendship."[3]

From the start, however, Evelyn was determined to keep up as much of her regular work and social schedule as possible. The country was celebrating "new" women, the ones who, in their teens and twenties, had watched (and often participated in) the women's liberation movements of the 1960s and 1970s. Now that group of twenty-two million was over forty-five years old. And it had become a most exciting target for advertisers, who gathered at an early 1989 panel discussion entitled "Age Power: Where the Money Is." The panel consisted of two magazine publishers, an advertising executive, and Evelyn, who would begin Dr. Norton's chemo cocktail soon afterward.

Five hundred and fifty eager marketers were in attendance at the iconic Pierre Hotel in New York to learn how to tap into the "new" women's aggregate household income of $729 billion ($2 trillion in today's money). Of course, that was right up Evelyn's alley. She spoke about the importance of women's self-image and of discipline when it came to diet and exercise, all of which were near and dear to her heart.[4] But now there were even more important points for her to make. No one in the room knew about her diagnosis; in fact, only a few people in her family knew about it. She was particularly careful to keep it from her eighty-five-year-old mother, so as not to worry her.

Evelyn was several months into treatment when she attended a March 22 breakfast meeting. Seated with her were Betty Ford, Ann Landers, Betty Rollin (a national television journalist who had written a book-turned-movie about her mastectomy), Kathleen Horsch (the American Cancer Society national board chair), and Dr. William Cahan (a thoracic and breast surgeon who had championed the anti-smoking campaign). The breakfast was to celebrate the launch of the Look Good, Feel Better program.[5]

Cancer never comes at a convenient time. When a woman is diagnosed, she might still have to work every day, care for her children, shop for essentials, and more, all while undergoing chemotherapy and radiation. It was no secret that many would experience hair loss (which also includes eyelashes and eyebrows) and skin problems from those life-saving treatments. Look Good, Feel Better—created jointly by the Cosmetics, Toiletries, and Fragrance Association and the American Cancer Society—aimed to provide services at cancer centers that would help women maintain a positive self-image.

They would be fitted for new wigs, courtesy of the ACS, and taught new ways to apply makeup with products donated by the association. Volunteers did the work, many of whom were cancer survivors themselves. It was a win for current patients, but it returned big benefits to the volunteers as well. They got a "helper's high," to use a term that had been coined just a few months earlier, in October 1988. It's the feeling of exhilaration and energy that comes from helping others. Research showed that the helper's high offered biological gifts as well. The release of feel-good hormones improves the body's immune function and lowers stress levels.[6]

The marketing panel, followed by the Look Good, Feel Better launch, were stepping-stones to an "aha" moment for Evelyn. For some time, she had been pondering how the family business could repay America's women. After all, they had loyally supported the Estée Lauder brands for over forty years. Donating makeup to Look Good, Feel Better was one thing, but Evelyn had a bigger vision.

She now knew firsthand the terror of breast cancer, with treatment that was, as Rose had said, "no piece of cake." Moreover, it seemed to Evelyn as though she spent her days tromping from one place to another: the doctor's office, the drugstore, the hospital, the physical therapy office. Locations were sometimes spread out over blocks, and even miles, in traffic-choked New York City. It was exhausting, on top of the exhaustion her chemotherapy was causing. Clearly, there was a huge hole in the system. And if her experience was difficult, Evelyn thought, what must it be like for those without her resources?

Creativity was part of her DNA, and she lit on an idea. She invited Dr. Norton over for a cup of tea, and, sitting at the family pinewood table in the kitchen, she began her pitch. A department store, Evelyn explained, is built around the customers' convenience. It allows them to buy a variety of things in just one place, with staff to help them find what they need within the store.[7] Using that as a metaphorical blueprint, why not do the same with a freestanding breast center? Rather than traveling all over town, everything a woman could need to combat and manage her breast cancer would be located in one place. In

1989, a single entity providing such comprehensive care was a totally novel, and brilliant, idea.

Dr. Norton loved it. And they wouldn't just offer state-of-the-art care. "We're interested in beyond state-of-the-art care!" he declared emphatically.[8] The two pooled their considerable strengths. He brought scientific and medical experience, and conceptualized his must-have list of what would be needed from a medical perspective. He also had strong leadership skills and a network of colleagues known for their work in breast cancer. That would be the pool he would tap into for staff members.

For her part, Evelyn's forté was fundraising and marketing. She now had decades of leadership experience at Estée Lauder, along with connections to the arts, industry, media, and government. She and Dr. Norton agreed from the start that the breast center couldn't be built on Lauder money alone. They wanted community buy-in, both figuratively and literally.[9] A small army of Estée Lauder staff members would work on organizing fundraising events and marketing them, along with the myriad other things a venture of this magnitude would need.

Not only would the center be one of a kind, it wouldn't be located on the MSKCC York Avenue campus. Rather, the property they chose on 64th Street was several blocks away from the bustle of the 565 patient rooms and more than 100 laboratories in the hospital. Their one-stop cancer treatment innovation would eventually become so successful, it would be copied throughout the world. But Evelyn and Dr. Norton were realists: there was a lot of money to raise before their dream of a serene port in the storm of breast cancer could become a reality.

—

Ohio congresswoman Mary Rose Oakar had met Rose Kushner shortly after arriving in Washington, D.C., in 1977. Rose had already testified before Congress on several occasions, garnering a number of congressional allies for breast cancer advocacy. But Oakar was different. Her sister had survived breast cancer, and the congresswoman was drawn so much to Rose's personality, she came to see her as a mentor. Together, they wrote a number of pieces of breast cancer legislation. (It was an unfortunate fact of congressional life that a dozen bills might be written on a topic before one was actually passed.)

And on September 18, 1989, they could see the goal line. That was the day Nevada representative Barbara Vucanovich introduced the Omnibus Breast Cancer Control Act, four bills aimed at improving access to early detection exams.[10] Like Rose, Vucanovich knew firsthand the importance of this work. Shortly after taking office in 1983, she had been diagnosed with breast cancer. And since her cancer had been caught through a screening mammogram, her motivation for the legislation couldn't have been greater.

The first act in the omnibus bill required Medicare to cover annual screening mammograms for women over the age of sixty-five. The next act required Medicaid to cover the screenings for women fifty to sixty-four. Third was a resolution targeting the twenty-six states that were, shockingly, still not mandating that private insurance companies cover the cost of mammograms. And finally, there was a bill requesting an increase in funding for educational pamphlets to inform women and their doctors about early detection.

By November 1, the bill had thirty-five sponsors.[11] A bill requires only one sponsor in order to be introduced, but the more who have signed on before discussions begin, the better. The congresswomen were working hard on their fellow legislators, but Rose had pages and pages of contacts at all levels in the breast cancer world who would put pressure on legislators. Each of those contacts had clout and more contacts. Rose was ready to cajole, argue, or beg—to do whatever was necessary—for help in getting the legislation over the finish line.

But where her spirit was willing, Rose's body was not. The cancer was gaining ground. A second metastasis appeared near the spot of the one she had found in 1982, and she underwent radiation for it. In 1989, a sarcoma appeared on her uterus and was removed by surgery. Again her medical team advised chemotherapy, and again Rose declined, stating there was no point going through the side effects just "to buy a few months."[12] The holidays passed and a new decade began.

In the first few days of 1990—to everyone's amazement—Rose was making calls from her hospital bed, urging support for the omnibus bill. It really shouldn't have been a surprise. From the time she had begun her breast cancer crusade sixteen years earlier, Rose was on the phone with *someone* seeking *something* from six-thirty in the morning until eleven at night.[13] Her "stubborn streak and loud voice" were her most powerful weapons until the end.

A winter morning sun peeked through clouds on Sunday, January 7. Its brightest rays must have appeared the moment Rose died, a testament to the light she had shown through her devotion to changing the breast cancer experience for all women.

Her many friends were quick to add their voices to the accolades that followed the announcement of her death. But admiration also came from those who hadn't always been allies. Dr. Bruce Chabner, who just a few years earlier had co-authored with Dr. Lippman the testy rebuttal to Rose's article about chemotherapy, said, "She is probably the single most important person in leading to this major change in breast surgery."[14]

Prior to her death, Rose had also been chosen to receive the 1990 James Ewing Award from the Society of Surgical Oncology (one of many awards she had received in her lifetime). Fifteen years earlier, the society's members had booed her as she spoke to them about breast surgery. "It's poetic justice," Harvey declared.[15] Rose had written a statement of thanks before she died, and he agreed to read it at their annual meeting in May.

Also fitting was the fact that Rose's obituary used the words "breast cancer" as her cause of death. Just a few years earlier, a death from any cancer was described as "a long illness" or with some other euphemism. Sometimes the newspapers simply pronounced that a person died, period. And of course, printing the word *breast* was a real taboo.

Not so for Rose. In fact, her cause of death was in boldfaced headlines: "Breast Tumor Kills Cancer Advocate," "Medical Writer Dies of Cancer," "Breast Cancer Fighter Dies of Disease." It was the first formal recognition of the illness Rose had fought both personally and publicly.

On Monday, January 22, journalist Margaret Mason began her tribute to Rose in the *Washington Post* with, "How could she, when there's still so much to do? Hadn't she taught us to stand up for ourselves? To dig in our heels and insist that we have a say in the big decisions?" The mock indignation was a beautiful echo of Rose's monumental achievements. Margaret ended with: "She gave us our voice. And now we cannot be quiet, not when someone dies of breast cancer every 13 minutes in the United States. And, not when we know that while 57,000 men died in combat in the Vietnam war, during that same 10-year period, 330,000 women died of breast cancer."[16]

Rose's name and legacy would live forever in many hearts, as well as in the records of Congress. On January 23, Mary Rose Oakar officially introduced the omnibus bill, now called the Rose Kushner Medicare Screening Mammography Act of 1990. It would wind its way through the congressional channels, ultimately becoming law on November 5.

The morning of January 30, a crowd began filling the Mazur Auditorium on the NIH campus. That had been the venue for the 1974 breast cancer presentation at which Rose's question prompted Dr. Bernard Fisher to admit there was no reason to remove pectoral muscles in a mastectomy. It had also been the venue of Rose's star performance at the 1979 Consensus Development Conference at which she successfully changed the status quo of a one-step mastectomy. It was the perfect place, then, for Rose's memorial. Harvey moderated, with eight individuals speaking of her vigorous, tireless, and courageous crusade for change, including her friends Mary Rose Oakar, Dr. Bernard Fisher, and Nancy Brinker.[17]

Two years after Rose died, medical historian Charles Rosenberg would write, "In some ways disease does not exist until we have agreed that it does, by perceiving, naming, and responding to it."[18] Breast cancer had been perceived and named before Rose Kushner, but it was her response to it that made all the difference.

⁓

Four and a half years earlier, on July 25, 1985, the towering, handsome leading man of more than sixty films, Rock Hudson, publicly announced to a shocked world in the form of a press release: "I have AIDS" (acquired immune deficiency syndrome).[19] On that day, Rose was no doubt still riding high from her *Phil*

Donahue Show appearance four months earlier. She would never live to see the impact that Hudson's relatively new disease would have on her ancient disease (which had first been recorded on papyrus around 2500 B.C.).

On June 5, 1981, the obscure disease that would come to be called AIDS was first mentioned in an article published in the weekly report from the Centers for Disease Control. The report discussed a sudden increase in diagnoses of a rare lung infection, pneumocystis carinii pneumonia, as well as an increase in the equally rare Kaposi's sarcoma. All of the patients were previously healthy, and all were gay men. As newspapers began picking up the story, the number of cases reported increased dramatically. By year's end, 337 men had been diagnosed, 130 of whom died (as compared to the 110,000 breast cancer diagnoses that year, with 37,000 deaths).[20]

Two men, Bobbi Campbell of San Francisco and Michael Callen of New York City, were among those diagnosed. Independently of each other, they began writing about their disease, the official name of which by this time had evolved from gay-related immune deficiency (GRID) to AIDS. While their personalities were completely opposite, the men's mission became united. "We must care about ourselves," Callen, with another New York activist, Richard Berkowitz, wrote, "obviously, others . . . do not care about us."[21]

Campbell and Callen recognized the importance of getting the word out about the disease's deadly track, both in their community and in the country at large. Rapid mobilization efforts were needed to find a cure and end the dying. Their campaign would not be a quiet one. They would take to the streets, loudly demanding research into the disease, as well as involvement in public health policymaking. And it worked. Fourteen months after the initial announcement about AIDS, two congressmen introduced pioneering legislation to allocate funds for research into the disease. And on May 18, 1983, the first AIDS bill, allocating $12 million to research and treatment, sailed through both houses of Congress.[22]

But that wasn't enough. Taking a page from Alice Wolfson and D.C. Women's Liberation, who rebelled at the Pill hearings, Callen and other gay New Yorkers crashed the National Lesbian and Gay Health Conference in Denver.

On June 12, 1983, they took the stage and read a document listing principles regarding how they wished to be treated, how to treat one another, and how to form caucuses to meet with media and government officials.

Called the "Denver Principles," the document became the Magna Carta of the AIDS movement. "We condemn attempts to label us as 'victims,' a term which implies defeat, and we are only occasionally 'patients,' a term which implies passivity, helplessness, and dependence upon the care of others. We are 'People With AIDS.'"[23]

The term *victim* was also frequently used in reference to those with cancer, and among that group it was also often met with equal scorn. Furthermore, like Rose's ongoing condemnation of the radical mastectomy, Callen's and Campbell's boldness shook the staid medical community. But not everyone was willing to "come out" with such bravado. Hudson had kept mum about his June 1984 diagnosis. As his disease accelerated, a thin, wan Hudson sought last-ditch hope in Paris at the Pasteur Institute, which had spearheaded AIDS research in France. It was from there that he announced his condition and, in doing so, his homosexuality. The latter had been a Hollywood secret for decades, as droves of women fell in love with him on both the big and small screens.

Like Shirley Temple Black, Hudson was much loved, and the first celebrity to publicly acknowledge this feared, fatal, and closeted disease. But there was one glaring difference. Unlike Shirley's announcement of breast cancer, when Hudson disclosed his disease, the resulting massive media coverage caused America to collectively and immediately decide something needed to be done.

Rock Hudson died on October 2, 1985, at the age of fifty-nine.[24] His courage to admit his illness and thereby his sexual orientation became his legacy. Suddenly the AIDS movement gained massive attention. Its cheerleaders came from all corners of humanity: gay and straight, the famous (Elizabeth Taylor had been Hudson's friend and confidant for three decades) and the unknown, those sick with the disease and those who hoped they would never see it.

And the money flowed. The day Hudson died, Congress allocated nearly $190 million more for AIDS research, $70 million over President Reagan's budget request for it.[25] The ever-loquacious Joan Rivers said, "Two years ago, when

I hosted a benefit for AIDS, I couldn't get one major star to turn out. Rock's admission is a horrendous way to bring AIDS to the attention of the American public, but by doing so, Rock, in his life, has helped millions in the process."[26] Between his announcement and the end of 1985, more than $1.8 million in private contributions was raised to support research and to care for AIDS patients. That was double the total collected in 1984.[27]

Private breast cancer donations never even came close to that number. After four years in operation, Nancy Brinker's Susan G. Komen Breast Cancer Foundation, then the country's premier breast cancer fundraising organization, had raised $1 million for research. (Brinker's dedication had become even more intense after her own breast cancer diagnosis and mastectomy in 1984.) And while AIDS diagnoses jumped by 89 percent in 1985, to 8,046, that figure was fifteen times lower than those who would be diagnosed with breast cancer the same year (119,000).[28]

The federal government's involvement in the AIDS movement accelerated as well. When the Institute of Medicine estimated in 1985 that $2 billion would be needed over the next decade for AIDS research and patient care, the gay community organized the AIDS Coalition to Unleash Power (ACT UP), bringing more attention, more advocacy, and more money to the disease.[29] *Time* magazine would call ACT UP's founders "the most effective health activists in history."[30] The organization pressed the government for additional funds; it demanded fast-tracked drug approvals and the creation of a federal Office of AIDS Research (an Office of Research on Women's Health wouldn't take shape until 1991).

And then, the cherry on top: the most famous woman in the world made a loud statement of support for AIDS patients and their movement. On April 9, 1987, Diana, Princess of Wales, was invited to London's Middlesex Hospital for the opening of their first dedicated AIDS ward. She stayed more than an hour, visiting with all ten patients, and was ultimately photographed shaking hands with one of them, without gloves.[31]

Certainly AIDS was a ghastly disease, with an alarmingly rapid progression and horrible mortality statistics. And while no one had the stomach to pit one disease against another, it was hard not to compare. Breast cancer had greater annual mortality numbers, and yet it was still underfunded, underresearched, and underdiscussed, with few celebrities voicing their indignation or even speaking about it since Shirley had fifteen years earlier. Not to mention the fact that no one had ever considered organizing a movement around a disease. Now there was a model. The growing army of breast cancer advocates took note of it all, collectively coming to realize that, as the AIDS activists had before them, they had to care for themselves.

By her own admission, Evelyn had lots of energy. "And energy breeds energy," she often said.[32] That was a good thing given the monumental task ahead of her in 1990. She had completed her own treatment, and fundraising for what would become the country's premier breast cancer center was marching steadily toward the $13.6 million goal. Evelyn and Leonard had gotten the ball rolling the previous year with a sizable personal donation, and she had even set up a satellite fundraising office within the hospital development office. Plus she had hired Susan Hirschhorn, former Metropolitan Opera development wizard, to helm their efforts.

Insomuch as Evelyn's employer, the Estée Lauder Companies, had been built on innovation, she brought that same philosophy to her endless fundraising ideas. She contacted major donors throughout New York City. She went to the media looking for support, either for publicity regarding the project or for a financial contribution. It was an easy ask since the company that bore her name was one of the largest spenders when it came to advertising and therefore wielded big clout. And as the breast center developed, she and her team sold hard-hat tours (or gave them as a thank-you for donations).[33]

It was important to both Evelyn and Dr. Norton that the moment a woman walked into the 40,000-square-foot center, she would see beauty. Norton called Evelyn a "design genius," saying, "We want to make it as de-medical as possible." That "design genius" was driven by her own experience. "When a person walks in, it may be with a degree of anxiety," Evelyn later said. "The whole idea is one of calmness, hopefulness, nurturing, embracing the patient."[34]

She envisioned smiling faces and enthusiasm to soothe the fear of patients as they were guided through the system. It was fear that had frozen Evelyn into inaction when she was first diagnosed. "Adding beauty and design to the breast center was obvious to me as a marketer," she explained. "It was never applied to a medical facility before." But Evelyn was accustomed to thinking outside the box.[35]

She used calm shades of beige and teal in the decor, wanting to complement the color scheme with art. But that presented a problem: fine art comes with a hefty price tag. It wouldn't look good to ask people to pony up big bucks for a breast center and then spend it on paintings. Again, Evelyn had a brainstorm.

Several years earlier, she had begun taking landscape photographs, uncluttered by figures. They had graced the Lauder holiday cards for the past ten years. Some of her favorite subjects were found around the Lauders' Aspen, Colorado, home, which sat on acreage surrounded by woods and a lake. She snapped pictures of the serene settings as she walked or cross-country skied. Others she took at their Putnam County house in upstate New York or on travels abroad. Why not incorporate them into the breast cancer center design? So she did. When all was said and done, nearly half of the more than six hundred photographs—some large and covering entire walls, others intimate and hung chairside—were Evelyn Lauder originals.

Meanwhile, Dr. Norton was focused on incorporating necessary technical things but not making them obvious. For example, the patient suites were much larger than a typical hospital exam room. That way, if a patient became ill, there was enough space for doctors and nurses to take care of her. More space also allowed for patients to have visits from a counselor, nutritionist, social worker, or psychologist even while they were receiving chemotherapy. "It's not just the disease we're attending to," he later said, "it's the whole person. So we pay attention to integrative medicine."[36]

And the clock was ticking. Their targeted opening date was summer 1992.

⟿

It had been described as "looking for a needle in a haystack."[37] However, on December 20, 1990, University of California, Berkeley, researcher Dr. Mary-Claire

King reported, "We're now at the point of knowing the handful of hay in which this needle lies, as opposed to having to search through the whole haystack." The "needle" she was referring to was the mutated gene she believed was responsible for inherited breast cancer. The road getting to this point had been a long one.

Born in a Chicago suburb in 1946, Dr. King majored in mathematics as an undergrad, and then planned to pursue a doctorate in statistics at UC Berkeley. A 1967 genetics course changed the entire trajectory of her PhD program—and the lives of millions of women. She was offered a postdoctoral fellowship at the University of California, San Francisco, in cancer epidemiology and genetics. She focused on breast cancer, intrigued by the notion that a pattern of breast cancers in families might be caused by a mutation.

Dr. King was ostracized for her genetic hypothesis, but she went back to the Berkeley campus and persevered. Still needing to earn a living while she researched, she applied for a tenured assistant professorship. Although universities were hiring more women, having them run their own lab was another thing. The head of the department made that clear: "I just want you to know you're only here because of these new regulations; we're really scraping the bottom of the barrel in hiring you." Dr. King wasn't deterred. "We'll see how long you feel that way," she told him.[38]

Seventeen years later, after Dr. King and her team had studied more than four hundred members of twenty-three families, who had had a total of 146 cases of breast cancer, they had narrowed down the location of the errant gene to chromosome 17. That was the handful of hay that led them to what they later called the *BRCA* 1 gene (named for the first two letters in the words *breast* and *cancer*).[39]

Interviewed about her discovery at the time, Dr. King had high hopes: "The long-term goal of this kind of work is to try to develop diagnostic techniques that will allow the detection of aberrant cells in the breast at an extremely early stage. Those cells could be removed and the woman go on with a normal life."[40] If such a thing were ever to become possible, what a wonderful gift for the 4 percent of families who are considered carriers of the mutation.[41]

Dr. King also applied her theory to the epidemic everyone was talking about in 1991. She was able to identify a genetic pattern of reduced susceptibility to AIDS. Two hundred thousand total cases had been reported in the United States since the disease had been identified nearly ten years earlier.[42] But with 175,000 breast cancer diagnoses in 1991 alone, it was hard to understand why that disease, too, wasn't considered an epidemic.

Sports, antiques, money, recreational vehicles, model railroading, computing, children, fashion, lifestyle: if there was a category for it, there was most likely also a magazine. And when publishing behemoth Condé Nast added *Self* to its family in 1979, they also added a new category: a woman's magazine with a twist.

"An extraordinary spirit and energy are emerging in women today. Fitness is the fuel." Phyllis Starr Wilson, the magazine's creator and founding editor-in-chief, was enthusiastically explaining the new platform. "We have acquired a strong appetite for the full experience of life—the exhilaration of the outdoors, the challenge and success of professional work, the honest enjoyment of sex. *Self* will be a guide to the vitality we need to do all the things we want to do."[43]

Phyllis had a history with Condé Nast, having previously been managing editor of the company's *Glamour* magazine. And insomuch as all of the Condé Nast magazines had offices in the same swanky Madison Avenue headquarters, Phyllis got to know Alexandra Penney, whose first job out of college was as an assistant editor at *Vogue*, another Nast holding. Alexandra left *Vogue* to earn a master's degree in fine art (she was also a gifted painter), but she kept a foot in journalism, freelancing while she painted. She stayed in touch with Phyllis, too, who would become a good friend and mentor. Shortly after Phyllis started at *Self*, Alexandra took an editorial position at *Glamour*, and the two women were once again working in the same building.

In 1979, statistics showed that one of every eleven women would be diagnosed with breast cancer at some point during her life.[44] Shortly after Phyllis took her position with *Self*, she became one of those statistics. Alexandra was shocked and disheartened. Phyllis kept working through surgery, chemotherapy, and radiation, but the disease tore relentlessly through her body. She stepped down from her position with the magazine early in 1987 and died of metastatic breast cancer at the age of sixty in 1988. Alexandra was devastated.

Two editors came and went at *Self*, each lasting just a year attempting to fill Phyllis's shoes. Then, in a stroke of sheer genius, in August 1989, Condé Nast named Alexandra as *Self*'s new editor-in-chief. She gratefully and reverently accepted, setting up her office at corporate headquarters in the very same space her friend had occupied for eight years.

Having been around magazines for decades, Alexandra was well aware of the true VIPs in the industry: the advertisers. As newspapers had spent the past decade consolidating, ads and money poured into glossy magazines. Each advertiser vied to have the first ad readers saw. Companies, particularly cosmetic companies, spent millions on full- or double-page all-color spreads at the front of fashion and lifestyle glossies. One of the largest spenders was Estée Lauder.

Although Leonard Lauder was the company president and Estée hadn't officially retired, the most prevalent personality was Evelyn. Perhaps it was because she was a Lauder, or perhaps because, as executive vice president, she'd shattered a glass ceiling or two. She was in charge of all of the company's new products and had become Estée's heir apparent in terms of being the most visible spokeswoman, a surrogate on the road now that the matriarch wasn't traveling as much. But in truth, Evelyn was incredibly pleasant, intelligent, knowledgeable, compassionate, and hardworking. Mostly she was just plain fun.

Consequently, Evelyn and Alexandra became acquaintances and then friends, frequently lunching at the 21 Club (often just known as "21") on West 52nd Street. The restaurant had begun life as a speakeasy in 1930, and it emerged after Prohibition as one of the hottest eateries in Manhattan. It had a very clubby feel about it. Nearly everyone who went there knew everyone else. And it was a particularly popular lunch spot among the city's well-knowns. Not surprisingly, that's precisely where Evelyn and Alexandra met for lunch on a lovely spring day in April 1991.

Evelyn was in full fundraising mode and shared her progress with Alexandra. The target date for the opening of the new breast center was just fourteen months away. Evelyn had suggested to fashion editors who were friends and had the ears of the country's women to write about the breast cancer epidemic. Most of them looked at her like she was crazy.[45] But Alexandra saw instantly what a brilliant idea it was. It would be too late to help Phyllis Wilson—of whom Alexandra thought nearly daily—but it could be a lifesaver for thousands of women in the future. As they chatted, Evelyn asked if perhaps an upcoming issue of *Self* could also feature a piece about the world-class center soon to be the gem of the city's medical offerings. That Evelyn had mentioned it was quite a coincidence, Alexandra said, as she was thinking about creating a breast cancer segment for the magazine. Running it in the October issue would be perfect, as that month had become the de facto "official" month for breast cancer awareness.

Prior to 1985, neither Evelyn, Alexandra, nor anyone else had contemplated the power of the word *awareness* when it came to breast cancer. But the ACS and Imperial Chemical Industries (maker of tamoxifen, now part of AstraZeneca) recognized that need and officially designated October 21–27, 1985, as the first National Breast Cancer Awareness Week.[46] They had given Betty Ford a starring role in the festivities and appointed her daughter, Susan Ford Vance (now Susan Ford Bales), the week's chair. On Tuesday, October 23, Susan testified, along with Rose, Nancy Brinker, and nine others, at a joint hearing in Congress.

"I am working on bringing this issue to the public front, to urge women to do all they can through early detection, not only to save their breasts, but their lives," Susan told the large group assembled in the Rayburn Office Building. "Breast cancer isn't like lung cancer, where in most cases, a woman chooses to be at risk. With breast cancer there are no choices but early detection."[47]

Understanding early detection and following through on it was the biggest challenge American women (and the men who loved them) faced. Understanding the *cause* of breast cancer was the biggest challenge American researchers faced. As Susan noted, in that era most lung cancers arose in smokers. And when other speakers before and after her spoke of the inequities in research funding and advances vis-à-vis AIDS, the point was brought up that the transmission of AIDS, too, had a behavioral component. Breast cancer's origins, however, remained a mystery.

In the ensuing years, breast cancer awareness weeks, and in some cases days, moved around the calendar, landing in nearly every month of the year. They were sponsored by hospitals, research universities, and even local ACS chapters. But with each passing year, a groundswell of events occurred in October. Eventually it became the unofficial breast cancer awareness month, and the first disease-related awareness month.

It was this evolution that had been the impetus for the casual conversation between Evelyn and Alexandra in April 1991. Before they left "21," however, the conversation had produced a road map that would forever affect breast cancer.

Chapter 11

~

Pink

"My pre-med adviser said to me that if I went to medical school, I would be killing some boy because he would have to go to Vietnam." Susan Love never shied away from telling a story, and always the whole story. She continued this memory with what her advisor had told her next: "'And you're just going to get the education, and then you're going to stay home and have babies, and it'll be totally wasted.'"[1] But Dr. Love wasted nothing.

She had always wanted to be a doctor, specifically a general surgeon. After completing her residency at Boston's Beth Israel Hospital, Dr. Love stayed on, becoming their first woman surgeon. As was the case with most female surgeons at the time, the only patients she saw were women with breast problems. Consequently, in 1988, she founded a breast center at the city's Brigham and Women's Hospital. Dr. Love and her all-female staff soon realized how little women knew about their own bodies. And it wasn't long before what had started for Dr. Love as a career in surgery transformed into a mission fighting breast cancer.[2]

Dr. Love had been born two decades after Rose Kushner, and they never met. Without missing a beat in 1990, however, she slipped easily into Rose's newly vacated position of dynamic breast cancer advocate. Dr. Love, too, agreed with the elimination of one-step and radical mastectomies. With relentless frequency, she questioned authority (exactly as Rose had), particularly doctors' automatic breast cancer treatment response of, as she called it, "slash, burn, and poison"—surgery, radiation, and chemotherapy—without considering other factors in a woman's life.[3] Dr. Love favored lumpectomies whenever possible and disagreed with aggressive chemotherapy and radiation.

In addition to their willingness to speak their passions at every opportunity, the two advocates shared a love of and skill for writing. In a replay of the medical community's outrage over Rose's book (a "piece of garbage," as one doctor had called it),[4] Dr. Love faced similar criticism when her *Dr. Susan Love's Breast Book* was published in June 1990.[5] Rose urged breast cancer patients to educate themselves before any treatment began. Dr. Love's book updated the progress made over the sixteen years between the two publications, thoroughly explaining the new beliefs about the disease and its most recent treatments. As Rose had, Dr. Love also wanted patients to be participants in what was happening to them. No surprise, then, that many of her colleagues (most of them men) hated her book, too.

The *Breast Book*'s publicity tour opened Dr. Love's eyes. On October 23, while speaking to the six hundred people filling the Salt Lake City Marriott's ballroom about the dearth of breast cancer research funding, she joked about organizing a topless march on the White House, adding "That should get President Bush's attention." When she finished speaking, dozens of women ran to the podium to ask if a date had yet been set for the march.[6] It made Dr. Love realize that there was a growing thirst for action.

Rose had advocated for a woman's right to choose when it came to treatment, frequently referring to her "streak of stubbornness and a loud voice" as her tools for getting things done. Dr. Love advocated a woman's right to live. She wanted research to focus on breast cancer's causes. To that end, she issued a call to arms: "Women, whether they're doctors or not, need to take to the streets, and yell and scream."[7] Those words resonated with women. While the breast cancer movement might have been conceived and gestated as a result of Shirley's and Rose's courage, it was officially born on Mother's Day, May 12, 1991.

The day was picture-perfect in Boston. Under a warm noon sun, seventy-five women gathered at the corner of Park and Tremont Streets to participate in an event organized by the Women's Community Cancer Project. Speeches were delivered, including one from Dr. Love, who shared the opinion that breast cancer—a disease that nearly always struck women—had not received adequate study. Funding decisions were being made by men, she said, and the time had come to not only increase the amount being spent (breast cancer received only $80 million of the well over $1 trillion federal medical research budget) but also decide *how* that money should be spent.[8]

Participant Rita Avitti agreed. "We want new ideas. We're tired of the same old research. . . . We're beginning to see this disease as a political issue." Rita, having been diagnosed with breast cancer in 1973, was spot on.[9]

Chanting "Save our mothers!" and "Save our lives!," the group left the pleasant corner of Boston Common and marched to the statehouse and then Government Center, ending at Faneuil Hall. With concurrent marches in Vermont and California, it was a preview of the larger meeting that would take place four days later, on May 16, in a Washington, D.C., law office conference room. There, Dr. Love spoke to the founders and members of breast cancer organizations from across the country, including the National Association of Breast Cancer Organizations (which Rose had helped found in 1986), Y-ME, the Women's Community Cancer Project, Can-ACT, the Mautner Project, and the Greater Washington Coalition for Cancer Survivorship.

The conference room had also been the destination of individuals who were eager to see change in the number-one health crisis for women. That was just one reason Fran Visco had come. In addition, she was a board member of the nearly twenty-year-old Philadelphia organization Women's Way. Part of the group's mission focused on women's health. Probably most important, the forty-three-year-old corporate litigator, wife, and mother had also been diagnosed with breast cancer three years earlier, at the age of thirty-nine.

Dr. Love was pitching the idea that the nation's numerous grassroots breast cancer organizations should come together under one umbrella. And she had a blueprint. Like the rest of America, she had watched the rapid spread of AIDS, the subsequent patient movement that was fostered by celebrities, and the astounding amounts of money flooding into labs for research on the disease. Furthermore, they were well organized. In 1984, the American Foundation for AIDS

Research (amfAR) was created, bringing together Dr. Mathilde Krim's foundation in New York and Elizabeth Taylor's foundation in Los Angeles. Dr. Love felt it was time to do the same thing for breast cancer.

The woman sitting next to Fran nudged her with an elbow. "She's famous," she whispered, pointing to Dr. Love, standing at the podium. "She wrote this unbelievable book."[10] During a break, another woman told Fran that the organization Dr. Love was suggesting was right up the lawyer's alley. Fran really didn't need the push; she had already made up her mind. She, like the other breast cancer advocates, had grown up in the age of movements: civil rights, anti–Vietnam War, abortion rights. Now she and the other women who had marched in the 1960s and 1970s were being diagnosed with and dying of breast cancer. She was in.

By the end of the day, the National Breast Cancer Coalition (NBCC) was official. The coalition's goals were clear: First, to increase research funding not just for treatments but to determine the cause of breast cancer. Next, to free up funds for underserved and uninsured women to gain access to care. And last, to increase involvement in legislative decision-making.[11] "Working the system" was something Rose had begun emphasizing as well in the year before her death. Just as the Denver Principles laid out the path for the AIDS movement, NBCC hoped their new organization would also become the "most effective health activists in history."

Before they parted, Dr. Love told the assembled group, "We have to be the voice, the obnoxious voice. We can't shut up now."[12] But to be that voice, breast cancer advocates had to learn the complicated—and sometimes mysterious—ways of American politics. Fortunately, they would soon collect a powerful and determined group of allies.

⁓

Becoming a congresswoman had not been on Pat Schroeder's to-do list before 1972, although she wasn't afraid of challenges. She had been one of fifteen women to earn a law degree from Harvard in 1964 (five short years after Ruth Bader Ginsburg had earned hers at Columbia).[13] A year earlier, Pat's husband,

Jim, had had a conversation with a friend considering a run for a congressional seat in their Colorado district. When the friend decided to pass, Jim asked if his wife would run. The friend replied, "What about yours?"[14] It was an unserious comment, but Pat (then thirty-two) took up the challenge with a platform of opposition to the Vietnam War.

Despite the Denver Democratic Women's Caucus endorsing her male opponent and the fact that many of the nation's other congressional races went to Republicans in the year of the Nixon landslide, Pat won. She was the first woman ever sent to Congress from Colorado. She was also the first woman appointed to the House Armed Services Committee. "When men talk about defense," Pat said shortly after her appointment, "they always claim to be protecting women and children, but they never ask the women and children what they think."[15] Her quick and barbed tongue became her trademark.

It was an era where few women ventured into the "good old boys" club of Capitol Hill. When a male colleague asked, "How can you be the mother of two small children and a member of Congress at the same time?" Pat replied without hesitating, "Because I have a brain *and* a uterus, and I use them both."[16]

In 1977, she and sister congresswoman Olympia Snowe, a Republican, co-founded and co-chaired the Congresswomen's Caucus (which in 1981 changed its name to the Congressional Caucus for Women's Issues). They focused on a litany of women's concerns, including discrimination and health. And while the women's movement certainly would have been aware of Pat's dedication, all of America learned her name in the 1990s. The country also learned that no cause, not even one as pressing as breast cancer, exists in a vacuum.

On September 10, 1991, Appellate Judge Clarence Thomas arrived at the Caucus Room of the Russell Senate Office Building. If the fourteen men of the Senate Judiciary Committee approved him, Thomas would become the next Supreme Court justice. There were no women on the committee; in fact, there wasn't even a women's restroom near the Senate chamber. At 10:05, committee chairman Joe Biden called the meeting to order. Thomas had already been thoroughly researched; over the next ten days, the committee would have the chance to see him onstage.

Several weeks earlier, Democratic committee staffers began to hear rumors of unsavory conversations between the judge and a woman who had once worked for him. The woman, however, did not want to come forward, preferring to keep her experiences buried in the past. The rumors were ultimately picked up by the FBI, which interviewed the woman three days after the nomination hearings had concluded. Her name was Anita Hill.

Once Pat and the rest of the women's caucus heard the story of Anita's sexual harassment and learned that Biden wasn't going to allow her to testify, they marched over to the Senate and demanded that she be heard. Pat advised Anita in advance of the hearing, and then escorted her to the hearing room on October 11. Pat was told she "could not come into the caucus because we were strangers."[17]

The questioning of Hill was insulting, capped off by a comment from Senator Arlen Specter. "You testified this morning . . . that the most embarrassing question involved—this is not too bad—women's large breasts. That is a word we use all the time. That was the most embarrassing aspect of what Judge Thomas had said to you?"[18] Specter neglected the context. Hill had alleged that Thomas had been describing a pornographic movie, which also included men with large penises and much more.

Hill had four supporting witnesses, none of whom were called during the three days she was questioned. The men on the committee aligned by brotherhood rather than politics, regarding Hill and her allegations with suspicion. Thomas was confirmed as a Supreme Court justice on October 15.

America's 129,055,067 women had watched the Thomas-Hill saga play out on their television screens.[19] Whether they believed all, some, or none of Anita Hill's testimony was only part of the story. The rest of it was the way she was regarded and treated by their senators. And that was the part they would remember at ballot boxes the next time they voted.

⟶

"Breast Cancer Report. Special editor: Evelyn Lauder."[20] The eleven pages that followed in the October 1991 issue of *Self* magazine were the fruit of the meeting

Evelyn and Alexandra had had at "21" in April. Dr. Norton was heavily quoted, his words filled with his signature optimism. "Many of us believe that we're now on the edge of totally curing breast cancer," he declared.[21] That might have been a stretch, but the outlook certainly looked more promising than in the past. According to the article, "Right now, physicians can cure ninety percent of patients with early-stage breast cancer."[22]

Not only was it the first time that a major glossy magazine devoted so much ad-free real estate to the disease, but there was an actual photo of a woman's breast, with a red circle around her lumpectomy scar. That procedure was explained, along with the latest on biopsies, mammograms, positive attitudes, and where to seek further assistance. And of course there was a piece featuring the new breast center project.

Throughout the preparation of the special section, Evelyn remained behind the scenes. She preferred it that way, although she did agree to being named special editor, and to the inclusion of a photo of her and Alexandra poring over a table stacked with paper. In the photo both sported sassy short hairdos; Evelyn's was a result of the regrowth of her hair after her chemo treatment, Alexandra's was styled in solidarity with her friend. Evelyn was of the opinion that the real story was the updates regarding all things breast cancer, which included Dr. Norton's continuing research and the exciting new center.

What a long way the world had come in the thirty years since Shirley Temple Black had shockingly revealed her breast cancer two decades earlier. Or had it? In 1991, one in nine women could expect to be diagnosed with breast cancer at some point during her life; that was a big jump from 1972's one in thirteen, when Shirley was diagnosed.[23] Furthermore, breast cancer was still considered a "woman's disease" by many and was therefore not pursued as rigorously as diseases affecting both genders.[24] And although the population was just about evenly divided along gender lines, men still held virtually all the power positions. Of the 100 U.S. senators, only two were women.[25] Among the House's 435 representatives, just twenty-eight were women.[26] Not surprisingly, then, women's health issues, including breast cancer, were rarely a funding priority. The situation was so glaring that Pat Schroeder exclaimed at a breast cancer event, "You can bet if I walked up to the Hill and told one of every nine men that he was going to lose a testicle this year, there'd be lots of research money!"[27]

The funding for breast cancer that year stood at a paltry $43 million (while $220.6 million was allocated for AIDS).[28] As Pat remarked at another breast cancer event, "They [her male counterparts] fund what they fear. They do not fear breast cancer, and they do not fear you."[29]

The government's disregard for women's health started at the top. When President George H. W. Bush was inaugurated in January 1989, he attempted to carry on what he and Reagan had done, including funding policies for AIDS. And as Reagan had done (despite the fact that his wife had had a mastectomy), Bush placed little importance on breast cancer. In fact, while he might have been a "genius" in foreign policy, he was "a fish out of water" on healthcare.[30] He disliked having to deal with it as much as he disliked broccoli.

However, the NBCC wasn't interested in the president's preferences, whether personal or political. They decided they would not be ignored by Congress any longer, and took aim at the breast cancer funding inequities. On June 13, 1991, they announced the launch of a letter-writing campaign called Do the Write Thing. The organization, now the umbrella for more than 160 breast cancer groups around the country, called for 175,000 letters to be written, one for each woman who would be diagnosed that year. The collection would be delivered to the president and Congress at the beginning of October.[31]

The letters' contents were completely up to the authors. Whether a letter writer copied the simple form letter the organization provided or composed a personal and powerful testimony, the overall goal was what was important: to motivate the United States government into action with regard to breast cancer research funding. The response was overwhelming. More than 600,000 letters arrived from women and men whose lives had been affected by the breast cancer epidemic. NBCC president Fran Visco proclaimed it "a testimony to the rage in this country over this issue."[32]

Taking a page from AIDS movement—that it was all about the optics—the NBCC organized a public event for Tuesday, October 8, in Washington, D.C.

Hundreds arrived in buses, from California to Florida and from Maine to Arizona. Women and men—some who had survived, some who were in treatment, some who would be dead in a year, some whose loved ones had already died—marched through the city from their gathering point and rallied on the lawn in front of the Capitol, joined by members of Congress, including Pat Schroeder and Mary Rose Oakar. There, beneath a brilliant blue sky, they held a press conference, poignantly punctuated by excerpts from some of the letters read out loud.

North Carolina resident Kathy Garraty wrote about her forty-year-old sister, whose breast cancer had metastasized to her brain before she died that January. "There was thick scar on the back of her head and neck from the removal of the tumor. . . . There was a hole in her neck to assist in breathing. Her breast was removed and a large scar remained across her chest. Her hair was gone from all the chemo. . . . No human being should suffer like this."[33]

Kathy was right. And yet every twelve minutes in 1991, a woman would die of breast cancer. And every three minutes another one would be diagnosed.[34] The words, and their writers, put a human face on the horrible disease. The event attracted media attention, as had the delivery of hundreds of boxes filled with thousands of letters to senators, representatives, and the White House. Now the question was whether or not any of it would have an impact on funding for breast cancer research.

⟜

"The tarnish on the American democratic ideal is that all too few citizens exercise the world's most cherished political power—the power to vote."[35] Three hundred and eight days after these words appeared in an editorial on January 1, 1992, Americans would vote for their next president. They would also vote for governors, mayors, judges, state officials, and U.S. senators and representatives. And the treatment Anita Hill had been given at the Clarence Thomas confirmation hearing was still very much in American women's memory.

Of the thirty-six Senate seats up for grabs, all were held by men. A full 435 seats in the House would be in play, all but twenty-eight of which were currently occupied by men. Suddenly, the men whose names would appear on ballots began looking for a woman-centric cause to support in an effort to garner women's votes. There were many in the breast cancer movement who could have given them some ideas. But, of course, they were never consulted.

By contrast with the male politicians, for Evelyn, breast cancer—and more specifically, the new breast cancer center—had consumed at least half of her time in one way or another every day since she and Norton had hatched the idea. She took a pause on March 3. Evelyn's eighty-seven-year-old mother, Mimi, had died. A kaleidoscope of memories poured forth: how she had clutched her little girl's hand in a desperate flight from the Nazis, survived imprisonment on the Isle of Man, and awakened her daughter so that the child could see the Statue of Liberty as they sailed past. Mimi was the architect of all of those moments. They defined the woman Evelyn had become.

Mimi never knew about Evelyn's breast cancer. The loving daughter feared it would worry her mother too much.[36] But Mimi was well aware of her daughter's quest to build the breast center. Her death now freed Evelyn from the fear she would find out. The family asked that, instead of flowers, donations to the center be made in Mimi's memory. And once she was laid to rest, the work had to continue.

Ever the savvy marketer, Evelyn went back to agreeing to be in the public eye as much as possible. Her name was mentioned—along with Barbara Walters, Rupert Murdoch, and Oscar de la Renta—as sporting a new Mephisto shoe style (although the word *style* is debatable). In another article, she was asked what item in her industry she couldn't live without if stranded on a desert island. "It would have to be sunscreen," she proclaimed.[37] And still another article described the dinner celebration for the 125th anniversary of *Harper's Bazaar*, hosted by her and Leonard at a New York restaurant, Mortimer's.[38]

On the surface, none of these opportunities for publicity appear connected to building a breast center. But Evelyn gambled that the more often her name was read or heard, the more likely people might be prompted to donate when asked. By April, they were incredibly close to the $13.6 million they needed. There was one more fundraising event on the schedule, and it was a biggie.

If your name is on millions of bottles of perfume and beauty products around the world, it isn't hard to imagine your path would cross with that of a princess. And that's exactly how Evelyn and Diana, Princess of Wales, came together for a London fundraiser. Diana was always game to use her celebrity for the causes dear to her, one of which was cancer; she was president of the Royal Marsden NHS Foundation Trust, a charity supporting Britain's premier cancer treatment center. Of course, the Royal Marsden foundation knew all about the MSKCC's breast center building project, and contacted their counterparts in New York with the idea of putting on a celebrity-studded event.

Susan Hirschhorn—who was heading the fundraising effort for the breast center—even moved to London for two weeks to make certain every detail was perfect. It would be a concert in tribute to the great Sammy Davis Jr., who had died of throat cancer two years earlier, at the age of sixty-four. It would feature big-name entertainers including Joan Collins, Lorna Luft, Tom Jones, and Jerry Lewis, plus the knock-it-out-of-the-park headliner, Liza Minelli. And it would be held at the iconic Royal Albert Hall in London. With American Express as the event's exclusive sponsor, Liza Minnelli's Tribute to Sammy Davis Jr. was ready for showtime.

When the curtain rose at 8:20 p.m. on Tuesday, June 23, 1992, the audience roared in delight after every unforgettable song and every sweet Sammy anecdote, each lovingly narrated by one of his friends. After the performance, the stars of the show waited patiently for Her Royal Highness to come meet them in the greenroom. "It's so much fun to perform for you!" Liza told Diana, giving her a big hug (they were good friends). Jerry Lewis, famous for hosting a muscular dystrophy telethon, joked, "We haven't had a job that paid us in years."[39] When everything was tallied, the Royal Marsden Cancer Appeal and MSKCC (the breast center was under its auspices) split $1.8 million.[40] Evelyn and her team had hit their goal, and gone beyond.

Over the course of history, when humankind contemplates a complex problem, it is not unusual for more than one individual to arrive at the same solution. In

1958, engineer Jack Kilby (age thirty-five) was a new hire at Texas Instruments in Dallas, while engineer Robert Noyce (age thirty-one) had just co-founded Fairchild Semiconductor in San Jose, California. Both men saw the need for a better type of circuit system and nearly simultaneously created the integrated circuit, which changed the world. A similar situation found its way to the breast cancer movement via Charlotte Haley's Simi Valley, California, living room.

Charlotte's grandmother had died of breast cancer at the age of forty-five. Her older sister was diagnosed with it in 1985, followed by her daughter in 1989. That's when Charlotte, a sixty-eight-year-old grandmother, drew the line. She was angry that no one seemed concerned about breast cancer's epidemic numbers, or the fact that only 5 percent of the National Cancer Institute's annual budget of $1.8 billion went to the disease.[41] In her eyes, it seemed that breast cancer had been "put on the back burner" and dismissed as a "women's disease."[42]

Decades later, there would hardly be an American who didn't have at least some awareness of breast cancer and the ways to prevent a death from it. Such was not the case in 1991. So that spring, Charlotte began hand-making peach-colored breast cancer ribbons (peach was her favorite color) and putting them in packets of five. Each packet was accompanied by a postcard, reading: "Breast Cancer Awareness Ribbon! Join this 'Grass Roots Movement.' Help us wake up the Legislators and America by wearing these ribbons. Not affiliated with any local, county, state, national, or federal organizations. (no donations solicited) For further information or ribbons, please call."[43]

The message ended with Charlotte's home phone number at the bottom. Her first ribbon distribution was at a meeting of her PEO (Philanthropic Educational Organization) Sisterhood chapter. The fact that all of the women wore her ribbons out the door gave Charlotte the courage to next pass them out in grocery store parking lots. Over the course of the year, Charlotte wrote to First Ladies Betty Ford, Rosalynn Carter, Nancy Reagan, and Barbara Bush. They didn't respond. But advice columnist Abigail Van Buren of "Dear Abby" fame (real name Pauline Phillips, twin sister to Eppie "Ann Landers" Lederer) did, writing back that she'd proudly wear the ribbon.

On the other side of the country, Alexandra Penney was at work designing *Self* magazine's 1992 October issue. As it had the previous year, the October issue would feature an in-depth breast cancer portfolio, including the latest developments in research and treatment, with a note about the opening of MSKCC's new breast center. Like Evelyn and others, Alexandra found the lack of attention to the increase in breast cancer diagnoses and the molasses-slow pace of research overwhelmingly frustrating.

A year earlier, a group of artists had come together to create a meaningful symbol for AIDS awareness: a red ribbon. The idea came from the yellow ribbons tied around trees as a reminder after hostages were taken at the American embassy in Iran in November 1979 (they were ultimately released in January 1981). The artist group called themselves Broadway Cares and made the ribbons to distribute to celebrities at the 45th annual Tony Awards. Actor Jeremy Irons put his on immediately and wore it throughout the televised event, of which he was the host.

New Yorkers began wearing them en masse as a show of solidarity for those affected by AIDS. Alexandra was no exception. While she was in the midst of pondering a similar emblem for breast cancer that would be equally influential and conspicuous, an executive editor ran into her office clutching a newspaper article. After a year of distribution, Charlotte's peach-colored ribbons had finally drawn press attention.

It was precisely what Alexandra had been looking for. She figured she and Charlotte were in similar boats. Both of them wanted better awareness for the unseen breast cancer epidemic, having watched people they loved suffer from it. It would be a perfect collaboration, and she called her immediately.

But after Alexandra had laid out her idea, Charlotte said no.[44] The magazine was too commercial, she thought, and would make money from someone else's pain. Simply put, she wanted nothing to do with them. Alexandra was dumbfounded. She explained that by bringing the ribbons to *Self*'s two million smart and caring readers, Charlotte would raise more awareness for breast cancer than she ever could on her own. That rationale fell on deaf ears, and the mild-mannered California grandmother promptly hung up on Alexandra.

By now, the clock for the magazine's layout was seriously counting down to press time. Alexandra, however, wasn't done. She consulted Condé Nast's legal team. They told her it was not possible to trademark an ordinary ribbon, and while the peach color might be contested, there was an entire rainbow to choose from. But which color? And how could it be worked into the magazine? Alexandra went to see "the big guy," Samuel I. Newhouse, then co-owner and chairman of Condé Nast, to ask about binding a ribbon of as-yet-undetermined color into the magazine's spine. The response: too expensive. What about a colored thread? Also too expensive.

Back in her office, Alexandra called Evelyn and asked to bring her an important idea. In minutes, Alexandra was headed to the company headquarters, along with the magazine's newly hired publisher, to outline her plan. At Estée Lauder's expansive counter space at the Manhattan Saks Fifth Avenue store, could they put ribbons in a glass bowl for customers to take?

"I'll do you one better," Evelyn told Alexandra without hesitation. "We'll put ribbons at *every* Lauder counter across the country!"[45]

All that remained was to choose a color, and there really was only one: pink. The color is a combination of red's passion and white's purity. It symbolizes nurture and compassion and evokes feelings of comfort and hope. Studies showed it had a calming effect.[46] In other words, pink was everything cancer is not. The color had come to be distinctively associated with women, too, just as breast cancer was distinctively associated with women. Pink had been the color on Alexandra's mind. And to Evelyn, the senior vice president of a cosmetics giant, one whose every product was packaged strategically, it was the best choice as well. Alexandra would handle the publicity, adding a pink ribbon graphic to the already finished pages of the magazine section. Evelyn would handle the manufacturing choices, selecting "150 pink" in grosgrain weave from the ribbon giant Offray.

Some of those same reasons for selecting pink might have been on Nancy Brinker's mind when she used it as a signature color for the Susan G. Komen Race for the Cure in 1990. Survivors received pink visors for the race that year, and pink ribbons the following year.[47] It was a lovely detail in the Susan G.

Komen Breast Cancer Foundation's large and growing portrait of breast cancer activism. Now, with the *Self* magazine/Estée Lauder plan, the pink ribbon would be front and center on a very large canvas.

In the ensuing years, there would be a great deal of discussion about who had the pink ribbon idea first, and whether its existence would help change the narrative about breast cancer. But that would be missing the point. Charlotte Haley, Alexandra Penney, Evelyn Lauder, and Nancy Brinker were all warriors fighting the same enemy. Since there had been little empathy for women with the disease, little research funding, and no awareness, wouldn't a combined effort better ensure change? And if a little pink ribbon could remind women of their risks, to do breast self-exams, to get mammograms, and to lobby for research funding in the face of a climbing number of diagnoses, wasn't that the success they all sought?

Nearly two hundred thousand Americans would be diagnosed with breast cancer in 1992.[48] That was more than 540 women every single day of the year—the equivalent of the passengers on one and a half jumbo jets flying into a dark abyss every single day of the year. And *that* infuriated Dr. Larry Norton.

"It's *cancer*, folks!" he proclaimed. "You're the Roman armorers and the Visigoths have knocked down the walls of the city and they are a block away from you and your family. Get with it, folks. It's *war!*"[49]

His analogy might have brought smiles to his audience of MSKCC doctors and staff. But its meaning was spot on. In a war against an advancing, brutal enemy, a good battle plan includes pulling in as many fighting assets as possible. The pink ribbon was one angle. Increasing research funding from the federal government would be equally critical.

After the emotional NBCC letter-writing campaign (which garnered media attention but not even a nod from Congress or the president), the organization determined they needed a more concrete approach. On a cold February morning in 1992, a day-long hearing convened in the Federal Ballroom of the Washington, D.C., Quality Hotel Capitol Hill. Fifteen titans of breast cancer research from institutions like Harvard, Yale, USC, Georgetown, and NIH made up the NBCC research task force. Nearly one hundred people—members of the coalition, journalists, women with breast cancer, and pharmaceutical company representatives—listened to them. There was no question that more money was needed. Their goal was to determine how much.

At five o'clock that afternoon, Harvey Kushner stood up to speak. It had been two years since Rose died, but she was certainly represented in his sage words.

"Across the hall there's another meeting. Across the street in another hotel, there's another meeting. And in each of those meetings there's a group of people talking about a different issue and the need for money. . . . Down the street from here are six hundred people, men and women, mostly men. These other people at these other hotels are going to be in their offices on Capitol Hill demanding their rights and they're going to get them."[50]

Forty million dollars had recently gone to a railroad museum in New Jersey. And $2.5 billion had just appeared in West Virginia's coffers because someone had lobbied for it.

"We've got to get our money before the Railroad Museum does. . . . teach women how to become politically active . . . so the next time we march on Washington we don't bring half a million letters, we bring a million. We don't have a few hundred women, we have a few hundred thousand. . . . Because that's the way the system works."[51]

Five months later, on July 29, 1992, "disease day" had come to Capitol Hill. Supporting funding increases for myriad conditions, including hearing loss, diabetes, dental research, and tuberculosis as well as breast cancer, were an assemblage of witnesses: doctors, organization leaders, patients, and NBCC's Fran Visco. Each witness was given three minutes to speak, timing for which was signaled by a light system on the senators' platform.

Fran had written her speech in her Philadelphia office. But on the train to D.C. she scrapped it for another, with a tone unheard of when cancer groups came to ask Congress for money. She was the final witness of the day.

"When the men in suits all but destroyed the savings and loan system in this country," she said, "the nation's economic stability was threatened and this Congress responded with billions of dollars.

"Because our cities are in danger of extinction, this Congress has found a way to appropriate emergency funds for the urban crisis.

"When this administration decided to wage a war, you found $7.5 billion to fund it.

"Women have declared war on breast cancer and you had better find a way to fund that war. . . .

"We will no longer be passive. We will no longer be polite. We can no longer afford to wait while Congress gets around to significant, decent funding for breast cancer.

"We implore you: you must find a way to appropriate the additional $300 million [the amount the task force recommended] for breast cancer research now. We can accept no less."[52]

The stunning declaration was followed by an equally stunning result. Breast cancer was personal to Iowa senator Tom Harkin; his two sisters had died of it. And as chairman of the Appropriations Subcommittee on Labor, Health and Human Services, and Education, he wielded the power to make inroads.

In 1991, he had shepherded a $25 million appropriation from the Department of Defense's (DoD) $3 billion budget. It was bound for the Army's Research, Development, Test, and Evaluation Program, "for the purpose of pursuing interservice research on breast cancer screening and diagnosis for military women and dependents of military men."[53]

Since the United States was not actively involved in any conflict at the time, where else but the DoD would one go for funds to declare a new war? Fran, Susan Love, and other members of NBCC sought him out as an ally.

On July 2, 1992, after much discussion and political wrangling, the bill spelling out Harkin's proposed appropriation of $210 million from the DoD for breast cancer research passed in the House of Representatives by a vote of 328 to 94. But the bill stalled in the Senate. Some senators argued that medical research money was in the realm of domestic programs and did not belong anywhere near the defense budget. But the majority of senators—the more farsighted ones—took a good look at the calendar.

In just weeks, a historic number of women would be running for office. That would no doubt energize and mobilize women voters. A no vote on breast cancer research funding would be an enormous slap in the face to half of every senator's constituents, many of whom were still stinging from the Clarence Thomas hearings.

When the Senate roll call vote occurred on September 22, the final tally was eighty-nine yeas and four nays, with seven senators notably not voting (including future vice president Al Gore and future vice president and president Joe Biden).[54] The Associated Press gushed that it was "the most generous federal financing yet for research into breast cancer." A nearly threefold increase in funding—totaling more than $400 million—would take effect in the next fiscal year, which began on October 1. The money would come from two sources: $210 million from the DoD and $196 million from the Department of Health and Human Services.[55]

The motivation of those who voted yes could be debated. But is that what really matters? As it was with the pink ribbon, isn't it more important to look beyond the lesser details and focus on the final result: the benefit to all those currently fighting the disease, and those who would be diagnosed in the future?

The final thrilling tally for 1992 would come on election day, November 3. After five women successfully won Senate seats and another forty-three won House seats, 1992 was officially dubbed the "Year of the Woman."[56] Having more women in government was a heady prospect. Perhaps it was truly a new dawn for American women. Perhaps women might also be elevated to top positions in other aspects of life. The thoughts called to mind the words Doris Day had sung decades earlier: "*Que sera, sera.* What will be will be."

Chapter 12

The Roaring Nineties

"Compliments on the photographs that have embellished her Christmas cards for the last 10 years or so have led Evelyn Lauder to offer [them] on a wider scale." The tiny article was buried deep inside a number of newspapers in September 1992. "The pictures she takes on travels . . . will go on exhibition Friday [September 11] through Sept. 19 at the Holly Solomon Gallery in Manhattan."[1]

Ultimately, Evelyn's showing would net $86,000 (over $190,000 today) for the breast center.[2] Although the construction funding goal had been met long before, the success of the exhibition taught Evelyn a valuable lesson about unique fundraising opportunities. Her hobby could become a force for good. In this moment, however, she would relish her dream coming true.

"The goal of this decade is to not only to find a cure for breast cancer, but to change, for all time, the way women with breast cancer are treated."[3] On September 30, 1992, the First Lady of the state of New York, Matilda Cuomo, had gratefully accepted the request to head up the dedication of the Evelyn H. Lauder Breast Center. As a longtime fighter in the war on breast cancer, Matilda was the perfect choice. And the recognition of Evelyn was so very justly deserved.

The breast center was billed as the nation's first to offer "not only state-of-the-art medical treatment but state-of-the-heart compassion as well."[4] This clever marketing position distinguished it from the University of California center that had opened in Los Angeles in June. Evelyn's breast center promised that any woman with a breast problem would be seen within forty-eight hours, and asymptomatic women seeking mammogram appointments would be screened within seventy-two hours. Given the anxiety that often accompanied *any* medical attention to a woman's breast, this was probably the most important line of all those written about the center.

A cascade of events followed the jubilant opening. On the heels of that important research funding vote on September 22, two days later Congress had officially declared October as National Breast Cancer Awareness Month, bringing everyone to the same page. That, in turn, made the October issue of *Self* magazine even more pertinent. A fourteen-page spread was evenly divided between the latest advances in gynecology and a complete update on research breakthroughs in breast cancer diagnosis and treatment. The image of a little pink ribbon, with its tiny gold safety pin, was on the cover and scattered throughout the breast segment.

Meanwhile, Evelyn had given her twelve thousand beauty advisors, patrolling the company's twenty-five hundred Estée Lauder counters across the country, their mission: disseminate 1.5 million pink grosgrain ribbons, along with cards reading, "I pledge my support for continued diligence in the battle against breast cancer."[5] This pioneering campaign brought breast cancer to the public—specifically women—in the safe and familiar world of cosmetic counters. Other entities, including hospitals, cancer organizations, and women's groups, jumped on the bandwagon, handing out their own handmade pink ribbons. The attention to the disease had a cumulative effect as it spread first in ripples and then in waves across the country.

Matilda Cuomo made one final point in her remarks, saying she hoped the breast center would carry the message "that women matter, that the diseases that affect primarily women matter, that the way in which women patients are treated matters most of all.

"Regardless of the illness, we must continue to do everything in our power to insure that all women are treated in a manner that upholds and encourages our dignity and our self-respect."[6]

Those hopes would take a while to materialize.

⬎

Over the previous one hundred years, members of the women's movement, including the women's health movement, had been referred to by disparaging labels such as "lunatic fringe" and "militant feminists."[7] Neither of those described Mark Nadel. In 1990, he was a fortyish, mild-mannered associate director for national and public health issues in the Government Accountability Office (GAO). And on June 18, he was testifying before the House Energy and Commerce Committee's Subcommittee on Health. As the investigative arm of Congress, the GAO had conducted an audit of the NIH. Nadel was there to report the discovery of a terrifying practice: the NIH was routinely excluding women from federally funded studies of drugs and other research projects.[8]

Furthermore, Nadel explained, the nation's (and the world's) premier research facility was knowingly making these exclusions in the face of a policy that forbade them to do so. Seven years earlier, in 1983, a task force had been created to look into women's health issues. The resulting report caused NIH—in 1986—to inform its research grant recipients that if women were not included in their work, the researchers had to provide the rationale for the gender bias. But nothing changed.

As a case in point, the results of the Physicians' Health Study were published in 1989. Over the course of five years, the practice of taking an aspirin every day had been studied to determine if it curtailed heart attacks. There were 22,071 men in the group. But no women were included, despite the fact that heart disease was the number-one killer of them, too.[9] Just as women's brains are different from men's, so are their hearts, lungs, and joints, something researchers ignored. Furthermore, pharmaceuticals don't act the same in women as they do in men, and diseases manifest themselves differently, too.

When Pat Schroeder and Olympia Snowe of the Congressional Caucus for Women's Issues uncovered women's exclusion from the aspirin study, they asked the GAO to start digging. That case was only the tip of the exclusion iceberg. Women were the fastest-growing group affected by AIDS, yet few women were included in any study. Phenylpropanolamine (PPA), the active ingredient in a popular diet aid, was tested on young men, despite the fact that middle-aged women overwhelmingly were the ones consuming the weight loss pills. There were many other examples, but probably the most shocking of all was a study exploring a connection between obesity and breast and endometrial cancers—and only men were included in that research project.[10]

In the few cases in which women were included in "gender-neutral" research, the vast majority of those studies did not report gender-specific findings. Female omission extended to animal studies as well. Typically, only male rats and males of other species were selected for study.

The money shortage had already been called into question with regard to breast cancer research, but it permeated all NIH work. Of the $7 billion the institutes received each year, only 13 percent was spent on women's issues.[11] Only three obstetrician-gynecologists were on permanent staff at NIH, causing one doctor to comment that NIH employed more veterinarians than gynecologists.[12] Basically, research was being done by white men, on white men, for white men. A majority of the scientific community had fallen back to the nineteenth-century premise that women were just smaller men, with a few anomalies.

Twenty-five centuries after Hippocrates announced his belief that the uterus was the key to all problems in women, his twentieth-century counterparts blamed hormones. Menstrual cycles—whether in human or animal subjects—would skew research results, they claimed. Testing females separately, or dividing out their results, would drive up the cost of research. In addition, testing pharmaceuticals on women who might be pregnant could have ill effects on the unborn fetus (although there was never any concern about potential danger to men's sperm).

In reality, women's reproductive years accounted for only about one-third of their lives. On any given day in 1990, there were millions of American women who were not susceptible to becoming pregnant. They had had hysterectomies, were menopausal, or were not sexually active. And if a signed informed consent was accepted for other things, such as X-rays, why wouldn't it be acceptable for clinical trials?

Nadel's 1990 report led to the 1993 NIH Revitalization Act, which mandated the inclusion of women in research, but did not mandate the analysis and publication of outcome data by gender. (Amazingly, that wouldn't happen until 2015.) But the lesson from all of this was clear: if the predominantly male research community and their predominantly male-led institutions weren't interested in including more than half of the population in their research, why would they be remotely interested in solving the mystery that was breast cancer? That would require some*one* and some*thing* special.

⁓

Most people would have seen the opening of the breast center as mission accomplished. But Evelyn wasn't most people. As she had watched her dream become a reality over the past twenty-four months, she had come to a crucial realization. While better care for those diagnosed with the disease was an important step, at the end of the day it was accelerated breast cancer research that would save lives. Without question, there were existing organizations that supported such research. Since its founding a decade earlier, Nancy Brinker's Susan G. Komen Breast Cancer Foundation had raised $10 million for screening, education, and research. It was an astounding amount for much-needed services, particularly in light of the federal government's anemic allocation from a much larger purse. And while the NCI focused on research, its layers of bureaucracy, combined with its lack of enthusiasm about studying women's cancers and its conservative approach to some projects it saw as outside the box, its breakthroughs were slow in coming to patients.

What the country—and the world—needed was a foundation with a laser-sharp dedication to breast cancer research and *nothing* else. It would be an entity willing to encourage and support projects and scientists with seemingly far-fetched ideas. After all, non-Halsted surgeries, chemotherapy, and lumpectomies had all at one time been considered heretical. Yet in 1992, those were all the norm. Lastly, it would embrace a goal the others didn't have: hastening the journey of research from lab bench to bedside.

Dr. Norton had similar unwavering beliefs about changes in research roll-out. "I think of myself as the March Hare," he once explained. "I like working underground amid the dark chaos of illness, helping my patients find their way out."[13] And like Evelyn, he knew that one of the best ways to help his patients out of that "dark chaos" was to help new ideas find their way out, too. Over the many months of working on the breast center with Evelyn, he watched her immerse herself in medical journals. Like Rose before her, she loved the science of it all, and what she couldn't understand on her own, Dr. Norton taught her.

Before the breast center even opened, they met again at Evelyn's kitchen table over tea. They had an extra $5 million from the center's fundraising, and they had already discussed the idea of a foundation. The agenda that afternoon was what shape it would take. Building on personal experience with his and Richard Simon's chemotherapy hypothesis years earlier, Dr. Norton felt that by granting seed money to reputable physicians and researchers, they could bypass the traditional medical institutions and government agencies that might consider some projects "too risky."

"Larry," Evelyn told him, "I've worked around creative people all my life. That's what we do. We create things. And they [creative people] need two things. They need freedom and they need security. You give them a job and let them run with it, knowing that failure is just a winding path that takes you closer to success."[14]

Their new foundation, therefore, would allow researchers the freedom to follow their most intriguing and inventive ideas. And it would give those researchers the security of knowing that even if they didn't find success, they wouldn't be out on the street because their grant wasn't renewed.

The funding process was another avenue Evelyn and Dr. Norton had to travel. The typical scientific grant request process was lengthy, cumbersome, and competitive. Complicated applications were submitted to be closely reviewed before decisions were made. Theirs would be a new and fresh process. As lovers of the New York art scene—and since both artists and scientists are creative people—they thought, why not build a program similar to artist grants?

The potential grantees would submit a straightforward, fifteen-page application. In the same way that members of an artist grant review panel attend performances and concerts and visit museums, therefore knowing the "scene," the breast cancer research panel would be scientific luminaries. They would have diverse expertise in multiple fields across the spectrum. And while Evelyn and Dr. Norton might have minimized the bureaucracy, the panel would still hold the grantees to high standards and require them to submit semiannual progress reports.

Two more points were non-negotiable for both of them. First, as they had done with the breast center, this would not be a Lauder project. Again, they wanted a broad base of support to demonstrate the foundation's legitimacy. And second, they didn't want to create an endowment fund, fearing it might someday curtail innovation. They would, however, continue fundraising to add to the $5 million seed money they already had. The name would make their mission unmistakably clear: the Breast Cancer Research Foundation (BCRF). And its mantra was simple and absolute: "A cure in our lifetime."[15]

Of course, having buy-in from wealthy donors would be crucial for the foundation to grow. To test the waters, Evelyn suggested a dinner party in her beautiful dining room, just a few steps away from the kitchen where they now sat. She would invite some of her friends, and Dr. Norton would assemble colleagues who were actually involved in cancer research, both in the laboratory and in the clinic. He envisioned that the dinner would illustrate a favorite quote from Quincy Jones, one of the greatest jazz musicians of all time: "You get the right people in the right room at the right time, and then you leave room for God to walk in."[16] God did. BCRF launched with six corporate partnerships.

After that discussion with Dr. Norton, but before she got too far down the road in the dinner party planning, Evelyn called her longtime friend and frequent sounding board, Myra Biblowit. Myra had a very personal connection to breast cancer. She was an only child, and her sister-in-law had become the sister she never had. The sister-in-law was diagnosed with breast cancer, and after her surgery was told it was early-stage. She was not given chemotherapy, which was the protocol of that era for early-stage disease. The very day the ACS reversed that opinion on chemotherapy, Myra's sister-in-law died of metastatic breast cancer. Myra remained convinced she might have lived had she been given further treatment.

Now, she listened to Evelyn explain the meeting she'd had with Dr. Norton, listing the pros and cons of creating a new foundation. Myra knew, however, that Evelyn had already made her decision when she concluded with, "I need another job like I need a hole in the head. But if I can do it, it would be a sin if I didn't."[17]

⁓

An economic boom was happening. American-style capitalism was pushing aside the sluggishness of the 1970s and 1980s. Job creation and technology innovation were going up, while inflation and poverty were going down. In the long run, productivity would exceed even that of the post–World War II boom. An air of youth returned to the White House on January 20, 1993, when forty-six-year-old William Jefferson Clinton moved in (along with his forty-five-year-old wife, Hillary Rodham Clinton), making him the third-youngest to do so. Furthermore, women were gradually filling positions in government and corner suites. The "Roaring Nineties" had arrived. And arriving with them came a new sector of business and economy: cause marketing.

Public awareness programs had risen and fallen in society's consciousness for centuries, with handbills nailed on hitching posts evolving into public service announcements playing out across television screens. But nothing rivaled the pink blizzard that appeared in the months following the ribbon's October 1992 debut. Six months after pledge cards were collected at Estée Lauder beauty counters, those cards made their way to the White House.

On May 13, 1993, First Lady Hillary Clinton welcomed Evelyn and Alexandra in the formal and famous Diplomatic Reception Room at the White House. As its name suggests, the room is most often used to welcome visiting heads of state. But given what accompanied Evelyn and Alexandria, the ground-floor room's proximity to the South Lawn entrance made it perfect for this event.

A large white steamer trunk was carried in after the women, emblazoned with the pink words "Wear this ribbon & make a difference." When the trunk was opened, a mound of more than a quarter million little pink missives appeared.[18] Each was from a woman asking that more federal funding be dedicated to breast cancer research. Evelyn's marketing sense guided her belief that it was important that the new president understood the growing grassroots support behind breast cancer research. She would also rely on the First Lady's predisposition to understand women's issues. It was already clear that Hillary Clinton would not be a figurehead; she would be involved and heard.

By this time, federal forms had already worked their way through the necessary channels to make the Breast Cancer Research Foundation an official 501(c)(3) nonprofit. Susan Hirschhorn, who had been at Evelyn's side throughout the campaign to build the breast center, had been named the foundation's first executive director. Since Evelyn and Norton expected that their grantees would come from a variety of locations, they had registered their nonprofit in all fifty states, allowing them to fundraise anywhere in the country.

With their nest egg in the bank, the BCRF review panel was already reading applications. And on September 21, 1993, they proudly launched "a significant new chapter in the crusade against breast cancer," as the founding press release read.[19] The first grant recipients represented eight institutions: Dana-Farber Cancer Institute in Boston; Vincent T. Lombardi Cancer Research Center at Washington, D.C.'s Georgetown University Hospital (Rose's home hospital); Mayo Clinic in Rochester, Minnesota; MSKCC's Evelyn H. Lauder Breast Center; Mount Sinai Comprehensive Cancer Center in Miami Beach; Swedish Medical Center Tumor Institute in Seattle, Washington; MD Anderson Cancer Center at the University of Texas in Houston; and the University of San Francisco.

The individual awards of $20,000 would allow researchers to carry out pre-clinical and pre-testing work on the causes and treatments of breast cancer, work that they hoped would validate their theories. Then, with proof in hand, the researchers could apply for larger government and private grants that otherwise would have been closed to them. Evelyn and Leonard hosted a dinner in their home to celebrate the inaugural recipients. The number of recipients grew so quickly, they would happily soon outgrow their dining room.

Press releases were sent from coast to coast. In one, Evelyn asserted, "With breast cancer predicted to kill 46,000 women in the United States this year, there is no greater enemy to challenge."[20] Each press release was also accompanied by the signature little pink ribbon, replicating the ribbon in the BCRF's logo.

Enlarging on the 1992 ribbon rollout, in October 1993, five thousand Estée Lauder cosmetic counters would be handing out three million ribbons at no charge, which Leonard and Evelyn donated personally.[21] Also available at the counter were breast cancer handbooks, produced by *Self*. If customers saw fit to donate $10 to BCRF, they could also take home an enameled pin version of the pink ribbon. Evelyn was adamant that her mission to bring awareness and funds to the breast cancer movement was completely altruistic, and evidence supports that claim. But this October, other companies would not be left out.

Avon announced that its representatives would also be selling pink ribbon pins, 415,000 of them, for $2 each.[22] The proceeds would benefit breast cancer education and prevention programs. Revlon was duplicating Estée Lauder's earlier pledge card program, partnering with NBCC to collect signatures at its counters. They would be presented to President Clinton with an appeal to make breast cancer a national health priority. (They ultimately collected 2.7 million.)

In fashion, Anne Klein and Company raised funds and awareness on behalf of a Long Island hospital. It was fitting, since Anne herself had died of breast cancer in 1974. Jones New York, Nine West, Oscar de la Renta, Ralph Lauren, Reebok, Hanes Hosiery, and others jumped in, raising money for a variety of entities. The industry's involvement prompted the former editor of a sample-sale newsletter to quip, "All these [fashion] companies' designers are dying of AIDS, but their shoppers are dying of breast cancer."[23]

She was right. The NCI had announced that breast cancer now struck one in eight women, and a staggering two and a half million American women currently had breast cancer (including one million who didn't know it).[24] With figures like that, it seemed that breast cancer had become the poster child for cause marketing. That made for an ironic chicken-and-egg situation.

A decade earlier, Rose had expressed disappointment that the women's health movement had been so disinterested in and silent about breast cancer. "Wherever women are, you go," she had admonished the movement leaders, pointing out that incongruous organizations often included women in their membership. "I would even reach out to the National Rifle Association, the Ku Klux Klan . . . and the Republicans, because regardless of their political thinking, they do have breasts. If it's truly going to be about women, it should be for all women."[25]

In reality, it was the army of breast cancer advocates (of which Rose was the generalissimo) who put a spotlight on the lack of attention to women's health. And that spotlight was far brighter and further-reaching than that of the movement itself. The Family and Medical Leave Act (1993), the Violence Against Women Act (1994), Offices of Women's Health at both the Food and Drug Administration and the Centers for Disease Control (1994), and the first guideline to include women's health issues in medical school curriculums (1996) all came about on the tails of the now ubiquitous pink ribbons. As it was in the discussion of the ribbon itself, the net result often outweighs the first to arrive onstage.

Nonetheless, it would still take years to change the language of breast cancer. While the surgeries were no longer spoken of as "mutilating," "disfiguring," and "maiming"—labels so terrifying that many women avoided the lifesaving operations—the media and public at large still had trouble shedding "cancer victim" and "cancer cure." In 1986, a fledgling group called the National Coalition for Cancer Survivorship (NCCS) addressed the former.

As it had been for AIDS patients, being a cancer "victim" suggested that a person was completely helpless in their situation, when in actuality, seeking treatment was very proactive. And at the time, being called a cancer "survivor" was predicated on a specific time goal line, generally five years of being cancer-free. But if the individual had a recurrence at five years plus one day, was the "survivor" title to be stripped away? The NCCS members refused to accept that. In creating their founding charter, they wrote, "From the time of its discovery and for the balance of life, an individual diagnosed with cancer is a survivor."[26] Case closed.

Addressing "cancer cure," however, was more challenging. While a better understanding of the disease had leaped light-years forward since Shirley's 1972 diagnosis, a pill to prevent or eradicate the disease remained elusive. Yet the breast cancer movement marched on.

⁓

"Turning her camera away from people and signs of cultural life, Evelyn Lauder has taken careful aim to celebrate nature season by season."[27] That description graced the inside flap of *The Seasons Observed,* a book of Evelyn's photography, released on September 6, 1994. It was by no means a vanity publication; on the contrary, it was the next logical step after her successful photography exhibit two years earlier. And, as with the exhibit, all proceeds would go directly into the BCRF coffers.

In addition, Evelyn—the woman with a million ideas—had added two new products to the Estée Lauder line in time for that October: Pink Ribbon All-Day Lipstick and Pink Ribbon Blush. The purchase of either would benefit BCRF. And just as education had permeated her career from the moment she went to work for the company thirty-five years earlier, she felt it equally important in the quest to slay the cancer beast. Every Estée Lauder counter was well supplied with breast cancer education pamphlets.

While Evelyn did indeed pour a great deal of mental energy into her fight against the disease, her day job was equally consuming. New products had to keep flowing, competitors had to be kept at bay, and marketing needed to be freshened up on a regular basis. The first company model, Karen Graham, who had also been the first model to ever have a beauty contract, remained the Lauder face for fifteen years.[28] They then began the practice of switching out models every five or six years. It wasn't because the women aged, but rather because "new" was the name of the cosmetics game. The current model had been in place since 1988; it was time for a quiet search to begin.

Meanwhile, in England, model and actress Elizabeth Hurley's life had been anything but quiet since May. She had been desperate to find a dress for the May 11, 1994, British premiere of *Four Weddings and a Funeral,* in which her boyfriend,

Hugh Grant, had a starring role. Although it was customary for designers to loan dresses to celebrities for such occasions, no one had heard of Elizabeth. Consequently, every call she made met with a resounding no. Then she called Versace, not yet a household name either. The manager in charge of loans at their flagship store on Old Bond Street was happy to loan Elizabeth something.

One might imagine that when one's beau is a star, prep for a premiere would involve a roomful of stylists. Such was not the case for Elizabeth, who did her own hair and makeup and then slipped into the borrowed dress. But this was not just any dress. It was black stretch silk that clung to Elizabeth's shapely body. It plunged down nearly to her waist from double shoulder straps and was slit up to the top of her left thigh. Most notably, the fabric was held together on either side by oversized gold safety pins in "strategical places." When she exited the car at the premiere, the press attention catapulted both Elizabeth and Versace into the headlines. Hugh Grant was only a minor detail in the news stories, and her dress became known as "*that* dress."[29]

On March 8, 1995, Elizabeth's "sculpted jaw and cheekbones, [and] blue-green eyes" officially became the fourth "face" of Estée Lauder.[30] This, despite her admission that she had been "gauche" when she first arrived in America: "At my first meeting with Estée Lauder, I had forgotten my hairbrush and had to borrow my friend's boots."[31]

After a full-scale press conference at the Royalton Hotel in New York, Elizabeth went to work, ultimately posing for every single product in the Lauder line. On her second day, Evelyn came to visit her at the photo shoot. Always keen to introduce something new when October rolled around, Evelyn asked Elizabeth if she'd be interested in helping with the breast cancer campaign. "Women all over the world are dying of breast cancer," Evelyn told her. "No one is talking about it and I want to change that."[32]

Of course, as the new model, Elizabeth would have had to say yes. But there was more that Evelyn never could have guessed. In 1992, Elizabeth's grandmother had died of breast cancer. The family didn't know much about her diagnosis or her treatment, and Elizabeth was convinced that her grandmother probably didn't know much about any of it, either. There was no question that she would help, and would be honored to be named "global ambassador" for Evelyn's enduring October concept: the Pink Ribbon Campaign. (It would later become known as the Breast Cancer Campaign.)

In 1994, *another* beautiful woman created *another* tsunami of publicity for wearing *another* black dress. On June 29, *Vanity Fair* hosted its annual summer party in support of the Serpentine Gallery, a free contemporary-art gallery in London's Kensington Gardens. Diana, Princess of Wales, was scheduled to attend, and the excitement over what she might wear had been building for days.

That also happened to be the date of a British television documentary entitled *Charles: The Private Man, the Public Role*. The prince had asked for the two-and-a-half-hour program, which had taken eighteen months to shoot and edit, and which would eventually be watched by so many in the United Kingdom that the country's electric utility, National Grid, reported a surge of power consumption during its airing. Among other topics, Prince Charles was hoping to garner some sympathy regarding his separation from Diana in December 1992.[33] That would require honesty, which would require admitting to infidelity. Thus, in the documentary, Charles admitted to having committed adultery.

It would have been completely understandable for the princess to skip the Serpentine party, to stay home until the news had settled down. But she did nothing of the sort. Forgoing the dress she had planned to wear (its design had been leaked to the press anyway), her final selection made jaws drop. When Diana exited her limousine, it was in a short, strapless black silk crepe cocktail dress. A chiffon train flowed in the wind behind her as she sailed to the receiving line. The dress also revealed her left thigh, and her black pumps elevated her height to over six feet.

To accentuate the dress, Diana had chosen a piece of statement jewelry. The seven-strand pearl choker, fastened with a duck-egg-sized sapphire nestled in two rows of diamonds, had been a wedding gift from the Queen Mother sixteen years earlier.[34] The princess never uttered a word about Charles's television bombshell. She didn't need to. Her smile, and what came to be called the "revenge dress," did the talking for her. It was "drop-dead" in more ways than one.

The dress took on even more importance when it made history again in June 1997 as lot number 2 in an unprecedented Christie's International charity auction. Months earlier, the now-divorced Diana complained to her eldest son, fourteen-year-old William, about how crowded all her dresses and gowns made her closet (although it wasn't so much a closet as a large room). William agreed and suggested, "Well, why don't you do something charitable with them?"[35] It was, Diana said later, "so appropriate and so simple!"[36]

Seventy-nine dresses, spanning the sixteen years she was Charles's wife, were selected. The proceeds would benefit AIDS charities in Britain and the United States, plus the Royal Marsden Cancer Center and the Evelyn H. Lauder Breast Center. Since the auction would be in New York, and since not only had Diana worked with Evelyn previously but the two had become friends, the planning committee began discussing elaborate, and expensive, party details fit for a princess. Evelyn, however, wanted as much money as possible to go to the charities.[37] After all, with the gowns as a backdrop, who needed decorations?

A 212-page catalogue went on sale before the auction. It was filled with information and designer sketches of the gowns, along with photos of the princess wearing them. Selling at $250 (nearly $550 today), it became a fundraiser itself, eventually raising $2.5 million when combined with syndication rights.[38] Diana thought it was better for her not to attend the auction, so as not to distract bidders. But she gladly attended the invitation-only reception the night before, where the dresses were on full display.

When Christie's International chairman Lord Hindlip welcomed bidders (he also served as auctioneer) the night of June 25, the frenzy began. There were no reserves, with the bidding on all items beginning at $5,000. For nearly three hours, the money rolled in. The "revenge dress" sold for $74,000. The "Elvis dress," a white silk crepe sheath with matching high-collared bolero jacket (both pieces of the outfit dripping in pearls and sequins) sold for $151,000. And the "Travolta dress"—an inky blue velvet off-the-shoulder number, so called because Diana wore it the night the actor had whirled her around the dance floor at a White House dinner—fetched a whopping $200,000.[39] Each purchaser also received a handwritten note from the princess on Kensington Palace stationery: "The inspiration for this wonderful sale comes from just one person. . . . my son, William."[40] It was simply signed "Diana," with the auction date.

When the dress and program sales figures were tallied, the auction cleared a record-setting $5.7 million, with the Evelyn H. Lauder Breast Center receiving a $1.2 million share (the equivalents of more than $11 million and $2.3 million, respectively, in 2024). Diana said afterward that wearing the gowns had given her pleasure, "particularly when representing my country abroad . . . I am extremely happy that others can now share the joy that I had wearing them."[41]

Like Evelyn, Diana was a mother before all else. She was always keen for her sons to see firsthand the joy of giving to others and of leaving a mark on the world. The sale must have been healing for Diana; clearing out her closet allowed her to move on from the fairy tale that never was. It was also the perfect segue into her new life.

But it would not be a long life. Sixty-seven days after that triumphant event, Diana, former Princess of Wales, died following a car crash in Paris. She was thirty-six years old.

⌢

"In my view, the more you speak about something, the more knowledge you have. And the more knowledge you have, the less fear you have."[42] Evelyn was firm in her insistence that all women needed up-to-date information about breast cancer. She continued the tradition of providing that information and other resources every October since that first *Self* magazine breast cancer section. In addition, her Pink Ribbon Campaigns included products whose proceeds went to BCRF, along with plenty of free pink ribbons fastened with little gold safety pins. By 1998, the company had educated women about breast cancer in more than forty countries.[43]

The sobering fact was that in the late 1990s, breast cancer research was still crawling along. Just one cent of every ten tax dollars collected was applied to the disease. Although Dr. Mary-Claire King refined her genetic research, and the biologic drug Herceptin (which targets cancer cells in the same way the body's own antibodies do) were brought to the public thanks to BCRF grants, the painfully slow advances were made worse by grim statistics. Breast cancer was the leading cause of cancer death for women between the ages of forty and fifty-five; more than 180,000 women would be diagnosed in 1998, and 43,500 would die.[44]

Whenever she could, Evelyn encouraged women to practice healthy living by curbing alcohol consumption, eating a diet low in fat and high in vegetables, exercising, and refraining from smoking. That lifestyle might not fully prevent cancer (it didn't for her), but a healthy body would at least be more capable of handling the disease. And even with her mother gone, Evelyn routinely deflected questions about her own diagnosis.

"My own situation doesn't really matter," she told a journalist. "The fact that I'm an activist is what's important."[45] She repeated that with finality, but also with a soft smile. Comparing herself to others wasn't Evelyn's style, but deep down she felt her cancer wasn't nearly as serious as other women's. So many had suffered much more. *Theirs* were the breasts she worried about. She fought against the disease on *their* behalf.

Evelyn really outdid herself in terms of awareness when the first October of the new century rolled around. On October 2, 2000, her Global Landmark Illumination Initiative would bathe landmarks around the world in pink lights as a reminder that breast cancer was still an epidemic. In 2000, 175,000 women in the United States alone would be diagnosed, a figure greater than the populations of Fort Lauderdale, Florida, Chattanooga, Tennessee, Syracuse, New York, or Ontario, California, the same year.[46]

Twenty-five landmarks in twenty countries were selected, including the Empire State Building in New York, Toronto's SkyDome, and Sydney's Museum of Contemporary Art. The illuminated structures were beautiful and moving sights. And the entire initiative would have made Evelyn's parents, Mimi and Ernst, so incredibly proud. What's more, all of her work had honored everything she had learned from them.

Her wonderful work ethic, building a loving family, expressing compassion for others—those were their gifts to her that she carried forward. But a single question had plagued Evelyn for decades: why had she been spared in the Holocaust when six million other Jews had perished? Had she known him, a Soviet neurologist could have given her an answer.

In 1974, the Soviet wrote to a British colleague who had suffered a near-death and life-crippling accident while hiking a mountain in Norway. "I am sorry it happened to you," the Soviet wrote to the Brit. "But if such a thing happens it can only be understood and used. Perhaps it was your destiny to have the experience; certainly it is your duty now to understand and explore."[47]

Evelyn's cancer diagnosis suddenly made it all crystal clear. Between those treated at the Evelyn H. Lauder Breast Center, the beneficiaries of medical breakthroughs (the research for which was funded by the Breast Cancer Research Foundation), the readers of the *Self* magazine articles and of all the other press she received, those who learned more about breast cancer via her Estée Lauder campaigns, and all those around the world who wore little pink ribbons, her work had gone on to save many, many women.

⌁

At the beginning of the twenty-first century, it was obvious that breast cancer was not just a medical problem. It had spread into politics, economics, industry, and society at large. It was discussed as much in laboratory settings as it was in corner offices. And yet, until a diagnosis became personal, "breast cancer" was just two words.

Shirley Temple Black, Rose Kushner, and Evelyn Lauder each made that discovery. All three women survived brushes with death in their early years, but even those didn't rock them as much as hearing the words "You have cancer." Standing at the dawn of the breast cancer movement, these three pioneers independently made decisions that forever changed the fortunes of others. And for that, the world is grateful.

Epilogue

When Estée Lauder died on April, 24, 2004, the world certainly lost an icon in the beauty industry. But Estée gave more to this world than cosmetics. If it hadn't been for her encouragement, along with that of Evelyn Hausman's father, a young couple who met on a blind date might never have married. What a hole that would have left in the breast cancer world if there had been no Evelyn Lauder.

Because of the success and reputation of the Evelyn H. Lauder Breast Cancer Center, she and Leonard helped build a new facility, which opened in 2009. Its sixteen stories on the MSKCC campus made it three times the size of the first center, but it maintained Evelyn's original vision of offering the best medical care within the framework of a beautiful, compassionate setting. And as she had also hoped, her "department store" concept in treating the whole woman was indeed replicated at major hospitals across the country.

Furthermore, Evelyn and Dr. Norton's amazing funding concept, the Breast Cancer Research Foundation, grew to proportions they never could have imagined. Since its creation in 1993, as of late 2024, total fundraising stands at more than $1 billion. And the foundation now funds over 250 researchers annually.[1]

Of all she did, however, Evelyn's greatest contribution to the nascent breast cancer movement was to create "awareness" of the disease. That word is tossed around without much thought today, but in the last decade of the twentieth century, breast cancer was not part of public consciousness. The government regarded it as a low-priority issue; the medical community often couldn't relate to its significance in a woman's life.

Evelyn was diagnosed with ovarian cancer in 2007. It was not a metastasis, nor was it genetic. After surgery and chemotherapy, she was proclaimed cancer-free, but it roared back in the summer of 2011. On November 12 that year, Evelyn died at home at seventy-five years of age, surrounded by those she loved.

The fifteen hundred people who attended her funeral two days later at Manhattan's Central Synagogue were a testament to her character, one of grace, charm, and extraordinary energy.[2] That night, after all the words about her incredible life had been written and spoken, the most visible and public memorial for Evelyn came from the Empire State Building, glowing in pink lights.

~

Although Rose had died (at the age of sixty) twenty-one years before Evelyn, she was still remembered as a much-revered voice in breast cancer among oncologists, researchers, advocates, and survivors. From her writing as a Jewish humorist to her hard-hitting books and articles, Rose's legacy was to audaciously take on the difficult topics. No one had ever written about breast cancer as she did, and that certainly became the biggest gem in her journalistic crown. Nor had anyone been as brazen as Rose was, taking on Congress, the NIH, the media, and sometimes even the public at large.

Fighting *for* birth control pill warning literature and mandated mammograms, her efforts continue to save lives today. Fighting *against* debilitating radical mastectomies and the psychologically damaging one-step procedure, her work still ensures that women have freedom of choice when it comes to the best route of treatment for themselves. While the "good old boys" medical establishment was not a forgiving one, Rose persevered, undaunted.

The breast cancer movement hadn't fully taken shape before Rose died. But she laid the groundwork, wielding her "streak of stubbornness and a loud voice" against anyone who stood in her way.

~

Although she would never shed her image as a child star, Shirley's government career took her to the heights she had hoped for, breaking through glass ceilings as she went. After she left her ambassador's post in Ghana in 1976, President Ford made her chief protocol officer. She finished her career as ambassador to

Czechoslovakia under President George H. W. Bush. Shirley was the country's first woman to hold all three of those positions.

When she was diagnosed with breast cancer, her courage to speak publicly accomplished three things. Using her celebrity, Shirley showed women everywhere that a breast cancer diagnosis wasn't shameful, nor did it need to be hidden. In addition, her hospital press conference confirmed that cancer certainly wasn't contagious. The scrum of reporters who showed up were proof of that. Most significant of all, Shirley was the first to suggest that women actually had treatment options. While it wasn't until Rose's dramatic 1979 performance at the NIH that the one-step protocol was officially declared to be unnecessary, Shirley had bravely begun that important public discussion seven years earlier.

A closet smoker, Shirley died of chronic obstructive pulmonary disease on February 10, 2014. She was eighty-five.

⁓

Shirley, Rose, and Evelyn never met. And they were certainly not alone in their advocacy of attention to breast cancer. There have been so many others, not the least of whom are Nancy Brinker, Fran Visco, and Dr. Susan Love (who died in 2023). To include all of those who deserve recognition in a single book would be an impossibility. Change often requires many people addressing the same problem, coming from different angles, at different times, with different solutions, but always with the single goal of improving the lives of others. Most importantly, these three radical sisters are proof of the quote often attributed to Margaret Mead: "Never doubt that a small group of thoughtful committed individuals can change the world. In fact, it's the only thing that ever has."

A generation ago, a book solely about women's health was a rarity in bookstores. Now there are entire sections devoted to the topic. Nor was breast cancer discussed a generation ago, let alone written about. But for the more than 310,000 women who will be diagnosed in 2025, for the more than 42,000 who will die from it in that year, and for the four million of us living in the United States who have survived the disease, this is our history.[3] Read it, share it, and be grateful for living in this era.

Acknowledgments

Hollywood has painted authors as invulnerable, intelligent, and intrepid. Sometimes we hover near that, but only with a team of caring individuals. And in writing this book, I was fortunate to have that team and more.

The archivists at the National Archives in Washington, D.C., provided great insight into congressional materials, while those at the Library of Congress chased down many newspaper and magazine articles. On the National Institutes of Health campus, the archivists at the Office of History and the librarians at the National Library of Medicine provided a wealth of historical treasures in the form of documents, videos, books, and photos.

Rose Kushner's expansive collection of papers resides at the Schlesinger Library on the History of Women in America, a part of the Harvard Radcliffe Institute. Many thanks to Jennifer Fauxsmith, research librarian, for leading me through the system and answering myriad questions while I was there, and afterward.

Family members and friends are crucial to painting the portrait of a biography subject, and those of these "radical sisters" were no different. Whether on the phone, via Zoom, or in person, my deepest gratitude to Tony Hausner, Leonard and Gary Lauder, Lesley, Gantt, and Todd Kushner, Barbara McLaughlin, Susan Hirschhorn, and Alexandra Penney.

When it came to questions about publishing, my dynamic duo consists of my brilliant agent, Dani Segelbaum, and my equally brilliant publicist, Lissa Warren. From phone calls of dismay to those of euphoria, thank you both so much for being there. The same goes for sister writer, Cindy Goyette.

My family has always been supportive, and I thank them for that. My brother, Chip Foster, has been particularly terrific in this endeavor. Not only was he supportive, but he hunted up even more newspaper articles than the Library of Congress.

And finally, to the man who has stood beside me, for better or worse, for fifteen years: David Martens, you are the best sounding board, cheerleader, dog walker, and husband a book girl could ever ask for.

Thank you all from the bottom of my heart.

Notes

Prologue

1. Quotes and descriptions from *The Phil Donahue Show*, March 18, 1985.
2. "New Cancer Survey Shows Progress in Understanding of Breast Cancer," National Institutes of Health press release, December 10, 1980.

Chapter 1

1. "Theodate Pope Riddle," Wikipedia, https://en.wikipedia.org/wiki/Theodate _Pope_Riddle, accessed November 20, 2024.
2. "Kickass Women: Theodate Pope and Belle Naish," *Smart Bitches, Trashy Books,* February 11, 2023, https://smartbitchestrashybooks.com/2023/02/kickass-women -theodate-pope-and-belle-naish/.
3. Aljean Harmetz, "Hollywood's Most Famous Child Star Tells in Her Own Words," *Town Talk,* October 30, 1988, https://www.newspapers.com/article/the -town-talk-child-star-1/146356594/.
4. "*The Blue Bird* (1940 Film)," Wikipedia, https://en.wikipedia.org/wiki/The_Blue _Bird_(1940_film), accessed November 20, 2024.
5. "Tiny Actress Dies From Flames," *San Francisco Examiner,* November 5, 1939, https:// www.newspapers.com/article/the-san-francisco-examiner-blue-bird-act /139391823/.
6. "CBS Studio Building," Wikipedia, https://en.wikipedia.org/wiki/CBS_Studio_ Building, accessed November 20, 2024.
7. Shirley Temple Black, *Child Star: An Autobiography* (New York: McGraw-Hill, 1988), 297–298.
8. "The Screen Guild Theater," Old Time Radio Downloads, https://www.oldtime radiodownloads.com/drama/the-screen-guild-theater, accessed November 20, 2024.
9. "Adolf Eichmann: Helps Vienna Jews to Facilitate Emigration (June 12, 1939)," Jewish Virtual Library, https://www.jewishvirtuallibrary.org/adolf-eichmann -helps-vienna-jews-to-facilitate-emigration-june-1939#google_vignette, accessed November 20, 2024.
10. Details of the Hausner family's application to exit Austria come from various historical documents, written in English and in German, provided by Evelyn's cousins, Tony and Kay Hausner.
11. Joseph Glatt, "Jews in Belgium," *Contemporary Jewish Record: Review of Events and Digest of Opinion,* edited by Abraham G. Duker, Vol. III, No. 4, July-August 1940. https:// www.bjpa.org/content/upload/bjpa/5_je/5_Jews%20In%20Belgium_July-August _1940.pdf.

12. "Imprisoned on the Isle of Man: Jewish Refugees Classified as 'Enemy Aliens,'" B'nai B'rith International, September 19, 2016, https://www.bnaibrith.org /imprisoned-on-the-isle-of-man-jewish-refugees-classified-as-enemy-aliens-html/.

13. David G. McCullough, ed., *The American Heritage Picture History of World War II* (New York: American Heritage Publishing, 1966), 99.

14. Leonard Lauder, *The Company I Keep: My Life in Beauty* (New York: Harper Business, 2020), 142.

15. Ibid., 143.

16. Ibid.

17. Isaac Rehert, *Looking In: An Autobiography* (n.p.: Isaac Rehert, 1992), 25.

18. Ibid.

19. Rose Kushner Oral History, Anne Kasper, interviewer, Kensington, MD, 1983, located at the Schlesinger Library, Harvard University.

20. Ibid.

21. Rehert, *Looking In*, 97.

22. Kushner Oral History.

23. "US Inflation Calculator," *Coin News*, https://www.usinflationcalculator.com.

24. Letter from Rose to Miss Shaffer, June 9, 1949, located at the Schlesinger Library, Harvard University.

25. Rehert, *Looking In*, 207.

26. Mark Finlay, "On This Day in 1949 an Air France Lockheed Constellation Crashed in the Azores," *Simple Flying*, October 28, 2022, https://simpleflying.com /air-france-lockheed-constellation-azores-crash-anniversary/.

Chapter 2

1. "New York City in the 1930s and 1940s—'If You Can Make It Here . . . ,'" We Refugees, https://en.we-refugees-archive.org/cities/new-york-city-in-the-1930s -and-1940s/editorial, accessed November 20, 2024.

2. Leonard Lauder, *The Company I Keep: My Life in Beauty* (New York: Harper Business, 2020), 144.

3. "Mrs. America: Women's Roles in the 1950s," *American Experience*, PBS, https:// www.pbs.org/wgbh/americanexperience/features/pill-mrs-america-womens-roles -1950s/, accessed November 20, 2024.

4. Melanie Hanson, "College Enrollment and Student Demographic Statistics," Education Data Initiative, last updated August 31, 2024, https://educationdata .org/college-enrollment-statistics; "Women's Education in the 1950s," *DesperateHousewives50*, May 8, 2012, http://desperatehousewives50.blogspot.com /2013/05/womens-education-in-1950s.html.

5. Lauder, *The Company I Keep*, 148.

6. Barnes & Noble advertisement, *Daily Sun*, September 14, 1954, 124.

7. Evelyn Lauder, unpublished memoir.

8. Lauder, *The Company I Keep*, 148.

9. "Estée Lauder," Cosmetics and Skin, September 20, 2023, https://cosmeticsand skin.com/companies/estee-lauder.php; advertisement in *New York Daily News*, December 9, 1923, 28, https://www.newspapers.com/article/daily-news-new-way -laboratories/142798977/.

10. Lauder, *The Company I Keep*, 5.

11. Ibid., 148.

12. Ibid.
13. James Sherwood, "Evelyn Lauder: Beauty Queen," *The Independent,* November 16, 2003, https://www.the-independent.com/news/people/profiles/evelyn-lauder-beauty-queen-78850.html.
14. Lauder, *The Company I Keep,* 148.
15. *Downton Abbey,* season 3, episode 5, 1:07.
16. Elizabeth Coman, *All In Her Head* (New York: Harper Wave, 2024), 229–231.
17. Christina Vanvuren, "The History of Hysteria: Sexism in Diagnosis," Talkspace, May 18, 2017, https://www.talkspace.com/blog/history-hysteria-sexism-diagnosis/.
18. Ada McVean, "The History of Hysteria," McGill University, Office for Science and Society, July 31, 2017, https://www.mcgill.ca/oss/article/history-quackery/history-hysteria.
19. *Downton Abbey,* season 1, episode 7, 6:30.
20. "Time to Start Thinking of Junior College Functions," *Baltimore Sun,* December 22, 1950, https://www.newspapers.com/article/the-baltimore-sun-baltimore-jr-college/143411566/.
21. "Student Recuperates, Earns Unusual Scholastic Record," *Baltimore Evening Sun,* December 6, 1950, https://www.newspapers.com/article/the-evening-sun-roses-appendectomy/124740663/.
22. Lesley Kushner, Zoom interview with the author, August 12, 2024.
23. Ibid.
24. Anne Edwards, *Shirley Temple: American Princess* (Guilford, CT: Lyons Press, 2017), 163–165.
25. "Shirley Temple Weds Sgt John Agar in Hollywood Church," *Boston Globe,* September 20, 1945, https://www.newspapers.com/article/the-boston-globe-shirley-wedding/139061866/.
26. "Shirley Temple Is Sure Her Husband, John Agar, Can Bring Home the Bacon," *Oakland Tribune,* February 16, 1947, https://www.newspapers.com/article/oakland-tribune-hes-a-natural/144238572/.
27. Shirley Temple Black, *Child Star: An Autobiography* (New York: McGraw-Hill, 1988), 444.
28. Ibid., 452.
29. "Shirley Temple Retires from Hollywood Scene," *Danville News,* December 21, 1950, https://www.newspapers.com/article/the-danville-news-shirley-retires/143832283/.
30. Black, *Child Star,* 495.

Chapter 3

1. "Text of Kennedy Speech," *The State,* July 16, 1960, https://www.newspapers.com/article/the-state-text-of-new-frontier/144757639/.
2. "Conclave Late in Starting," *Los Angeles Mirror,* July 16, 1960, https://www.newspapers.com/article/los-angeles-mirror-60000-at-coliseum/158599732/.
3. "United States—Population," CountryEconomy.com, https://countryeconomy.com/demography/population/usa?year=1960#:~:text=The%20female%20population%20is%20greater,of%20density%20population%20in%201960, accessed November 20, 2024.
4. "Women, Marriage, Education, and Occupation in the United States from 1940–2000," History 90.01: Topics in Digital History: U.S. History Through

Census Data, Dartmouth College, November 3, 2016, https://journeys.dartmouth
.edu/censushistory/2016/11/03/women-marriage-and-education-in-the-united
-states-from-1940-2000/.

5. Anne Walling, Kari Nilsen, and Kimberly J. Templeton, "The Only Woman in
the Room: Oral Histories of Senior Women Physicians in a Midwestern City,"
Women's Health Reports 1, no. 1 (2024): 279–286.

6. "History of Women in the U.S. Congress," Center for American Women and
Politics, Rutgers University, https://cawp.rutgers.edu/facts/levels-office/congress
/history-women-us-congress, accessed November 20, 2024.

7. "Prospects of Mankind with Eleanor Roosevelt; What Status for Women?,"
June 4, 1962, From the Vault, WGBH, https://openvault.wgbh.org/catalog
/V_285B9C3362534FFF8494B95922E3240B.

8. "Study Shows Women Still Slighted In Employment," *Charlotte Observer,* October
12, 1963, https://www.newspapers.com/article/the-charlotte-observer-no-need-for
-amend/145014745/.

9. Leonard Lauder, *The Company I Keep: My Life in Beauty* (New York: Harper Business,
2020), 152.

10. Mary Stanyan, "She's a Test Case for Beauty," *San Francisco Examiner,* November 10,
1970.

11. Pranay Gupte, "For Evelyn Lauder, the Past Is Certainly No Prologue," *New York
Sun,* October 3, 2005, https://www.nysun.com/article/business-for-evelyn-lauder
-the-past-is-certainly-no.

12. Lauder, *Company I Keep,* 193.

13. Ibid., 160.

14. Jane Lauder, "Notes from . . . Jane Lauder," Estée Lauder Companies (blog),
March 6, 2017, https://www.elcompanies.com/en/news-and-media/newsroom
/company-features/2017/notes-from-jane-lauder.

15. "Feminism," History.com, last updated April 8, 2022, https://www.history.com
/topics/womens-history/feminism-womens-history.

16. "Pregnancy Discrimination Act of 1978," U.S. Equal Employment Opportunity
Commission, https://www.eeoc.gov/statutes/pregnancy-discrimination-act-1978.

17. "The National Organization for Women's 1966 Statement of Purpose," National
Organization for Women, https://web.archive.org/web/20110902232426
/http://www.now.org/history/purpos66.html.

18. "Average Number of Children per U.S. Family (Historic)," PopulationEducation
.org, https://populationeducation.org/wp-content/uploads/2020/04/average
-number-children-per-us-family-historic-infographic.pdf, accessed November 20,
2024.

19. "Shirley Is Candidate; Says Country 'In Trouble,'" *The Times* (San Mateo, CA),
August 29, 1967, https://www.newspapers.com/article/the-times-shirleys-running
-2/145679175/.

20. "Shirley to Run for Congress," *Oakland Tribune,* August 29, 1967, https://www
.newspapers.com/article/oakland-tribune-shirleys-running/145679090/.

21. President Richard Nixon to Shirley Temple Black, November 8, 1961, Richard
Nixon Library, Yorba Linda, California.

22. "Shirley Is Candidate; Says Country 'In Trouble,'" *The Times.*

23. "McClosky Defeats Shirley Temple Black," *Redlands Daily Facts,* November 15, 1967,
https://www.newspapers.com/article/redlands-daily-facts-shirley-defeated
/145927584/.

24. "1968," Statistics, The American Presidency Project, https://www.presidency.ucsb .edu/statistics/elections/1968.

25. Tim Weiner, *One Man Against the World: The Tragedy of Richard Nixon* (New York: St. Martin's Griffin, 2015), 54.

26. Barbara Hackman Franklin, "President Richard Nixon: The Unlikely Champion of Advancing Equality for Women," June 2019, https://bhfranklin.com/wp-content /uploads/2019/06/President-Richard-Nixon-The-Unlikely-Champion-of -Advancing-Equality-for-Women-3-30-10.pdf.

27. Ibid.

28. "Shirley Says Declare War," *The Times* (San Mateo, CA), February 20, 1968, https://www.newspapers.com/article/the-times-shirley-says-declare-war /146373731/.

29. Robert Wiener, "Shirley Temple at the UN: Perfect Casting," *Newsday,* September 17, 1969, https://www.newspapers.com/article/newsday-nassau-edition-shirley -unschoo/146409247/.

30. Individual letters housed at the Richard Nixon Library, Yorba Linda, California.

31. "Miss Temple In U.N. Spotlight," *Troy Gazette,* September 17, 1969, https://www .newspapers.com/article/the-troy-record-rhinestones/158620730/.

32. "How Shirley Temple Black Went From Movie Star to U.S. Ambassador," *Newsweek,* April 9, 2018, https://www.newsweek.com/shirley-temple-went-movie -star-us-ambassador-876073.

33. U.S. Congress, "25th Anniversary of the United Nations: Hearings, Ninety-First Congress, Second Session, parts 1–2," 174, https://babel.hathitrust.org/cgi /pt?id=umn.31951p00820497q&seq=184&view=2up.

34. Marlene Simons, "'Lollipop' Mate Working Sailor with U.N. Crew," *Fort Worth Star Telegram,* March 22, 1970, https://www.newspapers.com/article/fort-worth-star -telegram-congressional-t/146838466/.

35. Claudia Kalb, "Shirley Temple Black's Remarkable Second Act as a Diplomat," *Smithsonian Magazine,* June 2022, https://www.smithsonianmag.com/history/shirley -temple-black-second-act-diplomat-180980038/.

36. "Sweden: American Delegate Shirley Temple Black Speaks at Closing Session of United Nations Environment Conference in Stockholm," British Pathé, June 17, 1972, https://www.britishpathe.com/asset/233634/.

37. Shirley Temple Black, "Don't Sit Home and Be Afraid," *McCall's,* February, 1973, 82.

38. Ibid.

39. Ibid.

40. Ibid.

41. Samuel Hopkins Adams, "What Can We Do About Cancer?" *Ladies' Home Journal,* May 1913, 21–22.

Chapter 4

1. "The 1970 March for Women's Equality in NYC," New-York Historical Society, March 10, 2015, https://www.nyhistory.org/blogs/march-for-equality-in-nyc.

2. Ellen Frankfort, *Vaginal Politics* (New York: Quadrangle, 1972).

3. "History and Legacy," Our Bodies Ourselves, https://ourbodiesourselves.org /history-legacy, accessed November 20, 2024.

4. Sandra Morgan, *Into Our Own Hands: The Women's Health Movement in the United States, 1969–1990* (New Brunswick, NJ: Rutgers University Press, 2002), 124.

5. Shirley Temple Black, "Don't Sit Home and Be Afraid," *McCall's*, February 1973, 82.

6. Ibid.

7. Ibid.

8. James S. Olson, *Bathsheba's Breast: Women, Cancer and History* (Baltimore: Johns Hopkins University Press, 2004), 62.

9. Ibid., 46.

10. Stefano Zurrida et al., "The Changing Face of Mastectomy (from Mutilation to Aid to Breast Reconstruction)," *International Journal of Surgical Oncology* 1 (January 2011), https://onlinelibrary.wiley.com/doi/10.1155/2011/980158.

11. Black, "Don't Sit Home and Be Afraid," 115.

12. Liz Smith, "Time Goes By at Le Cirque and Mortimer's," *New York Daily News*, October 21, 1988.

13. Black, "Don't Sit Home and Be Afraid," 116.

14. "From the Archives: President Nixon Signs the National Cancer Act," YouTube, posted by Richard Nixon Library, April 20, 2016, https://www.youtube.com/watch?v=lQYfC9kisHw.

15. Judith L. Pearson, *Crusade to Heal America: The Remarkable Life of Mary Lasker* (Rochester, MN: Mayo Clinic Press, 2023), 271.

16. "Shirley Temple Black Gives Press Conference After Cancer Treatment," British Pathé, 1972, https://www.britishpathe.com/asset/231985/.

17. President Richard Nixon to Shirley Temple Black, November 7, 1972, Richard Nixon Library, Yorba Linda, California.

18. Black, "Don't Sit Home and Be Afraid," 116.

19. Gerald Caplan, "An Outpouring of Love for Shirley Temple Black," *McCall's*, March 1973, 48.

20. Black, "Don't Sit Home and Be Afraid," 116.

21. Caplan, "An Outpouring of Love," 54.

22. "Fairbanks to Visit Dinah," *The Herald* (Rock Hill, SC), September 23, 1972, 17, https://www.newspapers.com/article/the-herald-us-soviet-pollution-talks-4-w/138314470/.

23. *Daily Oklahoman*, January 30, 1973, 8, https://www.newspapers.com/article/the-daily-oklahoman-shirley-on-dinah/146729301/.

24. *The Mike Douglas Show*, May 25, 1973.

25. *The Mike Douglas Show*, June 15, 1979.

26. "UM Graduates Urged Against Irrational Society," *Baltimore Sun*, June 4, 1972, https://www.newspapers.com/article/the-baltimore-sun-1972-u-of-m-commenceme/143615069/.

27. J. D. Hough to Rose Kushner, February 15, 1974, Schlesinger Library, Harvard University.

28. Carolyn Lewis, "Way to Victory Is Through the Heart," *Wilmington News Journal*, located in the Schlesinger Library, Harvard University.

29. Peter Lisagor, "The Housewife Who Went to War," *Chicago Daily News*, October 26, 1967.

30. Ibid.

31. Lewis, "Way to Victory Is Through the Heart."

32. Lesley Kushner, phone interview with the author, May 31, 2024.

33. Oral History of Rose Kushner, Anne Kasper, interviewer, April 6, 1983, located at the Schlesinger Library, Harvard University.

Chapter 5

1. Sara Alpern, "Helena Rubinstein," *Shalvi/Hyman Encyclopedia of Jewish Women*, https://jwa.org/encyclopedia/article/rubinstein-helena.

2. James Sherwood, "Evelyn Lauder: Beauty Queen," *The Independent*, November 16, 2003, https://www.the-independent.com/news/people/profiles/evelyn-lauder-beauty-queen-78850.html.

3. Pranay Gupte, "For Evelyn Lauder, the Past Is Certainly No Prologue," *New York Sun*, October 3, 2005, https://www.nysun.com/article/business-for-evelyn-lauder-the-past-is-certainly-no.

4. Leonard Lauder, *The Company I Keep: My Life in Beauty* (New York: Harper Business, 2020), 323.

5. Mary Burt Baldwin, "Childhood Occupations," *Chicago Tribune*, June 5, 1967, https://www.newspapers.com/article/chicago-tribune-adventure-playground/148254364/.

6. Ibid.

7. Gloria Biggs, "Cosmetics Queen Interviewed," *Press and Sun-Bulletin*, January 15, 1967, https://www.newspapers.com/article/press-and-sun-bulletin-estee-interview/148254631/.

8. Gupte, "For Evelyn Lauder, the Past Is Certainly No Prologue."

9. "Healthy Skin Is Clean Skin," *Democrat and Chronicle*, March 7, 1969, 16, https://www.newspapers.com/article/democrat-and-chronicle-healthy-skin-is-c/127137432/.

10. Winifred Care, "From a Beauty Cream, a Playground for Adventure," *Daily Telegraph*, July 20, 1970, 11, https://www.newspapers.com/article/the-daily-telegraph-evelyn-from-beauty-c/127138018/.

11. Ibid.

12. Lauder, *Company I Keep*, 4.

13. Rose Kushner, *Breast Cancer: A Personal History and an Investigative Report* (New York: Harcourt Brace Jovanovich, 1975), 3.

14. Delores Katz, "Breast Cancer Can Be Beaten," *Detroit Free Press*, January 13, 1975, 4, https://www.newspapers.com/article/detroit-free-press-breast-cancer-stats-1/148377870/.

15. "The Miss America Skit Gets Updated," *Newsday*, September 9, 1969, 70, https://www.newspapers.com/article/newsday-nassau-edition-bra-burning/145671742/.

16. "Bust Treatments," Cosmetics and Skin, last updated January 19, 2015, https://www.cosmeticsandskin.com/ded/bust.php.

17. Ibid.

18. Ibid.

19. Sandra Morgan, *Into Our Own Hands: The Women's Health Movement in the United States, 1969–1990* (New Brunswick, NJ: Rutgers University Press, 2002), 135.

20. Kushner, *Breast Cancer*, 3.

21. Ibid., 15.

22. Ibid., 7.

23. Ibid., 16.
24. Ibid., 13.
25. Wolfgang Saxon, "Dr. George Crile Jr., 84, Foe of Unneeded Surgery, Dies," *New York Times,* September 12, 1992, 10.
26. George Crile Jr., "A Plea Against the Blind Fear of Cancer," *Life,* October 31, 1955, 128.
27. Ibid.
28. George Crile Jr., *What Women Should Know About the Breast Cancer Controversy* (New York: Macmillan, 1973).
29. Kushner, *Breast Cancer,* 20.
30. Ibid., 22.
31. Ibid., 23.
32. Nan Robertson, "A Woman's Crusade Against 'One-Step' Breast Surgery," *New York Times,* October 22, 1979, 6.
33. Kushner, *Breast Cancer,* 24.
34. Ibid., 25.
35. Ibid., 26.
36. James S. Olson, *Bathsheba's Breast: Women, Cancer and History* (Baltimore: Johns Hopkins University Press, 2004), 39.
37. Ibid., 27.
38. Ibid., 18.

Chapter 6

1. Olga Khazan, "A Brief History of Contraception," *The Atlantic,* February 18, 2015, https://www.theatlantic.com/video/index/385602/a-brief-history-of-contraception/.
2. "Comstock Act of 1873," Wikipedia, https://en.wikipedia.org/wiki/Comstock_Act_of_1873, accessed November 20, 2024.
3. "Pills Given to 800," *Toronto Star,* June 14, 1960, 1, https://www.newspapers.com/article/the-toronto-star-pills-prevent-cancer/149214322/.
4. Planned Parenthood, "The Birth Control Pill: A History," last updated June 2015, https://www.plannedparenthood.org/files/1514/3518/7100/Pill_History_Fact Sheet.pdf.
5. Ibid.
6. "New Book Says Pill Ill-Conceived," *Indianapolis Star,* October 28, 1969, 9.
7. Statement of Elizabeth Connell, M.D., Hearings on the Present Status of Competition in the Pharmaceutical Industry, Before the Subcommittee on Monopoly, of the Select Committee on Small Business, U.S. Senate, 91st Congress, 1970, 6503.
8. Statement of Roy Hertz, M.D., Hearings on the Present Status of Competition in the Pharmaceutical Industry, Before the Subcommittee on Monopoly, of the Select Committee on Small Business, U.S. Senate, 91st Congress, 1970, 6029.
9. "History of Contraception," Birth Control Wisdom, February 18, 2015, https://birthcontrolwisdom.com/history-of-contraception/.
10. Statement of Philip Coffman, M.D., Hearings on the Present Status of Competition in the Pharmaceutical Industry, Before the Subcommittee on Monopoly, of the Select Committee on Small Business, U.S. Senate, 91st Congress, 1970, 6293.

11. "Alice Jacoby Wolfson '61," Barnard Alumnae, https://our.barnard.edu/s/1133/16/index.aspx?sid=1133&gid=1&pgid=5593#:~:text=The%20women's%20actions%20during%20the,of%20the%20women's%20health%20movement.

12. Rose Kushner Oral History, Anne Kasper, interviewer, Kensington, MD, 1983, located in the Schlesinger Library at Harvard University.

13. Rose Kushner to Mr. Michael, August 19, 1974, Schlesinger Library, Harvard University.

14. Betty Ford, *The Times of My Life* (New York: Harper Collins, 1978), 182.

15. Ibid., 184.

16. Rose Kushner, *Breast Cancer: A Personal History and an Investigative Report* (New York: Harcourt Brace Jovanovich, 1975), 310.

17. Rose Kushner to Pat Sweeting, October 2, 1974, Schlesinger Library, Harvard University.

18. Judy Flander, "Rose Kushner Made Her Own Decisions About Breast Cancer," *The Missoulian,* September 4, 1974, 28, https://www.newspapers.com/article/the-missoulian-conversation-with-friedma/150981180/.

19. Kushner, *Breast Cancer,* 20.

20. "Betty Ford Enters Hospital for an Exam," *Morning Herald* (Hagerstown, MD), September 28, 1974, 1, https://www.newspapers.com/article/the-morning-herald-betty-ford-1/149386455/.

21. Kushner, *Breast Cancer,* 312.

22. James Wieghart, "First Lady Called OK After Cancer Surgery," *New York Daily News,* September 29, 1974, 2, 17, https://www.newspapers.com/article/daily-news-fouty-quotes/149671445/.

23. Kushner, *Breast Cancer,* 43.

24. "Dramatic New Findings in Breast Cancer Research," *Nevada State Journal,* September 30, 1974, 2, https://www.newspapers.com/article/nevada-state-journal-dramatic-new-findin/149708907/.

25. "Breast Cancer Report to the Profession Suddenly Is a Report to the Nation; Treatment Progress Noted," *Cancer Letter,* October 4, 1974, https://cancerhistoryproject.com/tcl-archive/19741004-1/.

26. "Survival Rate Is Linked to Post-Surgery Drugs," *Waterloo Region Record* (Ontario, Canada), October 1, 1974, 50.

27. "Surgery Like First Lady's Might Offer No Advantage," *Nevada State Journal,* September 30, 1974, 2.

28. Kushner to Sweeting.

29. "Doctor Optimistic About First Lady's Recovery," *Simpson's Leader-Times,* October 1, 1974, 2, https://www.newspapers.com/article/simpsons-leader-times-bettys-recovery/149719464/.

30. Stanley Johnson, "ACS Breast Clinics Booked Months Ahead," *Lawton Constitution,* November 20, 1974, 29, https://www.newspapers.com/article/the-lawton-constitution-switchboards-bus/149723849/.

31. Ford, *Times of My Life,* 186.

32. Rose Kushner, "What If It's Cancer," *Washington Post,* October 20, 1974, 1.

33. Rose Kushner to Jerry, October 7, 1974, Schlesinger Library, Harvard University.

34. Rose Kushner to Dr. Thomas Dao, October 7, 1974, Schlesinger Library, Harvard University.

35. "Helen Reddy's 'I Am Woman' Tops the Charts," Jewish Women's Archive, December 9, 1972, https://jwa.org/thisweek/dec/09/1972/helen-reddy.

36. Rose Kushner Oral History, Anne Kasper, interviewer, Kensington, MD, 1983, located at the Schlesinger Library, Harvard University.

37. "Happy Rockefeller's Breast Removed," *Longview Daily News,* October 17, 1974, 1, https://www.newspapers.com/article/longview-daily-news-happys-mastectomy/149721873/.

38. Cass Vanzi and Harry Stathos, "Rocky's Wife to Lose Second Breast," *New York Daily News,* November 25, 1974, 3, 30, https://www.newspapers.com/article/daily-news-happys-second-mastectomy/148687440/.

39. Robert Joffee, "On the Good Ship Lollypop," *Times Colonist,* September 16, 1974, 5, https://www.newspapers.com/article/times-colonist-about-shirleys-appointme/149897512/.

40. Darius S. Jhabvala, "Nixon, Brezhnev Pledge New Ties for World Peace," *Boston Globe,* June 19, 1973, 1, https://www.newspapers.com/article/the-boston-globe-the-soviets-and-waterga/149967172/.

41. Jane E. Brody, "If Detected Early, Breast Cancer May Be Cured," *Courier Journal,* November 19, 1972, 131, https://www.newspapers.com/article/the-courier-journal-95-find-their-tumor/149972193/.

42. Gerald Caplan, "An Outpouring of Love for Shirley Temple Black," *McCall's,* March 1973, 52.

43. "Alcoholics Anonymous," Wikipedia, https://en.wikipedia.org/wiki/Alcoholics_Anonymous, accessed November 20, 2024.

44. Kushner, *Breast Cancer,* 147.

Chapter 7

1. *Jaws* (film), Wikipedia, https://en.wikipedia.org/wiki/Jaws_(film)#Marketing, accessed November 20, 2024.

2. Stanley Meisler, "Men Dominate Opening of Women's Conference," *Los Angeles Times,* June 20, 1975, 1, https://www.newspapers.com/article/the-los-angeles-times-un-conference-on-w/150436044/.

3. Ibid.

4. Samuel Gregory, *Man-Midwifery Exposed and Corrected,* 1848, https://dohistory.org/archive/doc041/041_title_img.html.

5. Stacy Weiner, "A Brief Timeline of Women in Medicine," Association of American Medical Colleges, 2024, https://www.aamc.org/news/brief-timeline-women-medicine.

6. Evan Jenkins, "Women in Medicine Up Sharply," *New York Times,* July 17, 1974, 77.

7. Rose Kushner, *Breast Cancer: A Personal History and an Investigative Report* (New York: Harcourt Brace Jovanovich, 1975), 190.

8. Ibid., 175.

9. Ibid., 191.

10. "How's Shirley Doing?," *Macon Telegraph,* September 1, 1975, 5, https://www.newspapers.com/article/the-macon-telegraph-hows-shirley-doing/150930446/.

11. Judy Flanders, "Cancer Patient Writes Book on Breast Cancer," *Ames Tribune,* September 24, 1975, 10, https://www.newspapers.com/article/ames-tribune-description-of-book/150989828/.

12. Kushner, *Breast Cancer,* xii.

13. Flanders, "Cancer Patient."
14. Dolores Katz, "Breast Cancer Can Be Beaten," *Detroit Free Press,* January 13, 1975, 4, https://www.newspapers.com/article/detroit-free-press-breast-cancer-stats-1 /148377870/.
15. Rose Kushner Oral History, Anne Kasper, interviewer, Kensington, MD, 1983, located at the Schlesinger Library, Harvard University.
16. Quotes from this and all following notes Rose received are part of her papers at the Schlesinger Library, Harvard University.
17. Lesley Kushner, email to the author, May 30, 2024.
18. "Examination on the Treatment of Breast Cancer, What Treatment Is Best, Where Physicians Differ and the Risks and Costs Involved," Before the Subcommittee on Health, of the Committee on Labor and Public Welfare, United States Senate, 94th Congress, 2nd Session, 1976, 1.
19. Ibid., 2.
20. Ibid., 3.
21. Ibid., 24.
22. Ibid., 11.
23. Kushner, *Breast Cancer,* 236.
24. Ibid., 255.
25. Ibid., 246.
26. Ibid., 207.
27. Ibid., 254.
28. Ibid., 256.
29. Ibid., 211.
30. Ibid., 324.
31. "The National Cancer Program," Before a Subcommittee of the Committee on Government Operations, United States House of Representatives, 95th Congress, 1st Session, 1977, 441.
32. Ibid., 1.
33. Ibid., 449.
34. Ibid., 447.
35. Rose Kushner Oral History.

Chapter 8

1. Advertisement in *The Morning Call,* November 19, 1978, 114, https://www.news papers.com/article/the-morning-call-breast-surgery-ad/151867428/.
2. "Breast Form Evolution," Amoena, https://www.amoena.com/us-en/about-us /breast-form-evolution/, accessed November 20, 2024.
3. Cynthia Martens, interview with the author, January 17, 2024.
4. Judy Klemesrud, "Woman Files Suit to Recover Costs of Breast Rebuilding," *New York Times,* August 3, 1979, 12.
5. Judy Klemesrud, "Women's Rights to Surgery Insured," *Daily Breeze* (Torrance, CA), January 27, 1980, 45.
6. Rose Kushner, *Alternatives: New Developments in the War on Breast Cancer* (Cambridge, MA: Kensington Press, 1984), 282.
7. Glennys McPhimimy, "Women Get Information on Breast Cancer Too Late," *Sunday Camera* (Boulder, CO), August 20, 1978, 25.

8. Kushner, *Alternatives*, 133.
9. Ibid., 134.
10. Rose Kushner to Judge Thomas Platt, February 3, 1978, located at the Schlesinger Library, Harvard University.
11. Kushner, *Alternatives*, 175.
12. Ibid., 177.
13. Ibid., 178.
14. National Institutes of Health Consensus Statements, "The Treatment of Primary Breast Cancer: Management of Local Disease," June 5, 1979, https://www.ncbi .nlm.nih.gov/books/NBK50809/.
15. Rose Kushner, "Mastectomy No Longer Automatic," *Baltimore Sun*, July 6, 1979, 17, https://www.newspapers.com/article/the-baltimore-sun-the-right-to-choose /151872206/.
16. Sascha Cohen, "This Is What Breast Cancer Activism Looked Like Before the Pink Ribbon," *Time*, October 17, 2016, https://time.com/4531239/breast-cancer -activism-history/.
17. Ibid.
18. Ibid.
19. Judith Randal, "Mastectomy and Radical Decisions," *New York Daily News*, June 10, 1979, 84, https://www.newspapers.com/article/daily-news-randal-article-re-rose /144947060/.
20. Handel Reynolds, *The Big Squeeze: A Social and Political History of the Controversial Mammogram* (Ithaca, NY: ILR Press, 2016), 18.
21. Ibid.
22. Ibid., 19.
23. Judith Randal, "Breast Cancer Testers May Halt X-Ray Use," *New York Daily News*, July 15, 1976, 238, https://www.newspapers.com/article/daily-news-nci-test-under -scrutiny/152334169/.
24. "Experts Seek End to Mammography," *Press and Sun-Bulletin*, July 15, 1976, 35, https://www.newspapers.com/article/press-and-sun-bulletin-bailar-quote/152333859/.
25. Reynolds, *The Big Squeeze*, 24.
26. "Women at Cancer Unit Split on X rays," *Press and Sun-Bulletin*, August 1, 1976, 62, https://www.newspapers.com/article/press-and-sun-bulletin-nci-women-divided /152334413/.
27. Kushner, *Alternatives*, 156.
28. Ibid., 157.
29. Jimmy Carter Presidential Files, Office of Staff Secretary, Folder 3/26/80, Container 156, Vol IX-A, page 66, https://www.jimmycarterlibrary.gov/sites /default/files/pdf_documents/digital_library/sso/148878/156/SSO_148878_156 _02.pdf.
30. Rose Kushner Oral History, Anne Kasper, interviewer, Kensington, MD, 1983, located at the Schlesinger Library, Harvard University.
31. Ibid.
32. Ibid.
33. Rose Kushner, "Recurrence," unpublished manuscript written for *Outlook*, November 9, 1982, located at the Schlesinger Library, Harvard University.
34. Rose Kushner Oral History.
35. Kushner, "Recurrence."

36. Rose Kushner Oral History.
37. Lesley Kushner, Zoom interview with the author, November 20, 2023.
38. Kushner, *Alternatives,* xxii.
39. Ibid., xxiii.
40. Koen D. Flach and Wilbert Zwart, "The First Decade of Estrogen Receptor Cistromics in Breast Cancer," *Journal of Endocrinology* 229, no. 2 (May 1, 2016), https://joe.bioscientifica.com/view/journals/joe/229/2/R43.xml.
41. Kushner, *Alternatives,* xxvi.

Chapter 9

1. Nancy G. Brinker, *Promise Me: How a Sister's Love Launched a Global Movement to End Breast Cancer* (New York: Crown Archetype, 2010), 196.
2. Ibid., 143.
3. Ibid., 191.
4. Ibid., 192.
5. Ibid., 198.
6. Yuning Wang, "Chemotherapy's Hidden Origins," Drug Discovery News, September 26, 2023, https://www.drugdiscoverynews.com/chemotherapy-s -hidden-origins-15763.
7. In this discussion, for oncology, see B. J. Kennedy, "Origin and Evolution of Medical Oncology," *Lancet* 354 (December, 1999): 41; on nursing, see Helene Brown, "Where We Were and Where We Are Going," *Clinical Journal of Oncology Nursing* 16, no. 6 (December, 2012): 555.
8. Sharon Batt, *Patient No More: The Politics of Breast Cancer* (Charlottetown, PEI: Gynergy Books, 1994), 97.
9. Rose Kushner, "Is Aggressive Adjuvant Chemotherapy the Halsted Radical of the '80s?," *CA: A Cancer Journal for Clinicians* 34, no. 6 (1984): 345.
10. Ibid.
11. Ibid., 346.
12. Baron H. Lerner, "Ill Patient, Public Activist: Rose Kushner's Attack on Breast Cancer Chemotherapy," *Bulletin of the History of Medicine* 81, no. 1 (2007): 230.
13. Ibid., 233.
14. Marc Lippman and Bruce Chabner, "To the Editor," *CA: A Cancer Journal for Clinicians* 35, no. 3 (1985): 186, https://acsjournals.onlinelibrary.wiley.com/doi/epdf/10.3322 /canjclin.35.3.186-a.
15. Ibid., 188.
16. Quotes and descriptions from *The Phil Donahue Show,* March 18, 1985.
17. Rose Kushner Oral History, Anne Kasper, interviewer, 1983, located at the Schlesinger Library, Harvard University.
18. Barron H. Lerner, *The Breast Cancer Wars: Hope, Fear, and the Pursuit of a Cure in Twentieth Century America* (New York: Oxford University Press, 2003), 3.
19. Ellen M. Goudsmit, "All in Her Mind! Stereotypic Views and the Psychologisation of Women's Illness, in *Women and Health: Feminist Perspectives,* ed. Sue Wilkinson and Celia Kitzinger (Bristol, PA: Taylor & Francis, 1994), 10.
20. Sandra Morgan, *Into Our Own Hands: The Women's Health Movement in the United States, 1969–1990* (New Brunswick, NJ: Rutgers University Press, 2002), 120.
21. Goudsmit, "All in Her Mind," 7.

22. Andrew M. Colman, *A Dictionary of Psychology* (New York: Oxford University Press, 2015), 441, https://books.google.com/books?id=UDnvBQAAQBAJ&pg=PA441#v =onepage&q&f=false.

23. Cate Lineberry, "Martha Mitchell: The Socialite Turned Watergate Whistleblower," History.com, April 25, 2021, https://www.history.com/news /martha-mitchell-watergate-kidnapping.

24. Rose Kushner's Memorial, National Institutes of Health, January 30, 1990, Schlesinger Library, Harvard University.

25. Ibid.

26. Margaret Mason, "'Race for the Cure': Carrying on the Spirit of Rose Kushner," *Washington Post,* January 22, 1990, https://www.washingtonpost.com/archive /lifestyle/1990/01/22/race-for-the-cure/d81cf671-f03f-4d8d-b012-af79b633250e/.

27. Rose Kushner's Memorial.

28. "Nancy Reagan Undergoing Tests for Breast Cancer," *Baltimore Sun,* October 17, 1987, 12, https://www.newspapers.com/article/the-baltimore-sun-nancy-advocates -mastec/158839907/.

29. Associated Press, "Some Doctors Disagree on Choice of Surgery," *Boca Raton News,* October 18, 1987, 5, https://www.newspapers.com/article/boca-raton-news-nancys -over-the-top-sur/153216566/.

30. Susan Baer, "The Biggest Problem Is Fear," *Baltimore Sun,* October 20, 1987, 3, https:// www.newspapers.com/article/the-baltimore-sun-rose-on-nancy-pt-2/153217130/.

31. James Sherwood, "Evelyn Lauder: Beauty Queen," *The Independent,* November 16, 2003, 36, https://www.the-independent.com/news/people/profiles/evelyn-lauder -beauty-queen-78850.html.

32. Leonard Lauder, *The Company I Keep: My Life in Beauty* (New York: Harper Business, 2020), 243.

33. Ibid., 242.

34. Ibid., 246.

35. Gary Lauder, interview with the author, August 4, 2024.

36. Lauder, *Company I Keep,* 333.

37. Ibid., 334.

Chapter 10

1. Ronald Piana, "An Aspiring Musician Changes Course and Becomes a Breast Cancer Specialist Who Makes Music: Larry Norton, MD, FASCO," *ASCO Post,* June 3, 2019, https://ascopost.com/issues/june-3-2019-narratives-special-issue/an -aspiring-musician-changes-course/.

2. Charles Schmidt, "The Gompertzian View: Norton Honored for Role in Establishing Cancer Treatment Approach," *JNCI: Journal of the National Cancer Institute* 96, no. 20 (2004): 1492–1493, https://doi.org/10.1093/jnci/96.20.1492.

3. Susan Hertog, "A Cosmetics Queen Builds an Anti-Cancer Empire," *Philanthropy Roundtable,* Fall 2018.

4. Elaine Boies, "Older Women Beginning to Attract Attention of the Fashion Industry," *Town Talk,* January 17, 1989, 17, https://www.newspapers.com/article/the -town-talk-every-and-older-fashion/152204098/.

5. Liz Smith, "Time Goes By at Le Cirque and Mortimer's," *New York Daily News,* March 19, 1989, https://www.newspapers.com/article/daily-news-look-good-feel -better-foundi/132848351/.

6. David R. Hamilton, "Helper's High," May 7, 2015, https://drdavidhamilton.com /helpers-high/.

7. Larry Norton Oral History, Breast Cancer Research Foundation, September 26, 2023, https://www.bcrf.org/blog/bcrf-2023-podcast-larry-norton-breast-cancer-30 -years/.

8. Evelyn H. Lauder Breast Center of Memorial Sloan-Kettering Cancer Center Press Release, 2009, National Museum of American History, Smithsonian Institution.

9. Susan Hertog, "The War Against Breast Cancer: The Physician and the Lady," *Philanthropy Roundtable*, Fall 2016, https://www.philanthropyroundtable.org /magazine/the-war-against-breast-cancer/.

10. "House Legislators Sponsor New Breast Cancer Bills," *JNCI: Journal of the National Cancer Institute* 81, no. 21 (1989): 1609, https://academic.oup.com/jnci/article -abstract/81/21/1609/938317?redirectedFrom=fulltext.

11. Ibid.

12. Barron H. Lerner, *The Breast Cancer Wars: Hope, Fear, and the Pursuit of a Cure in Twentieth Century America* (New York: Oxford University Press, 2003), 259.

13. Lesley Kushner, Zoom interview with the author, December 5, 2023.

14. "Rose Kushner, 60; Medical Writer, Advocate," *Los Angeles Times*, January 13, 1990, 177, https://www.newspapers.com/article/the-los-angeles-times-rose-obit-poetic /143604276/.

15. Ibid.

16. Margaret Mason, "Race for the Cure: Carrying on the Spirit of Rose Kushner," *Washington Post*, January 22, 1990, https://www.washingtonpost.com/archive /lifestyle/1990/01/22/race-for-the-cure/d81cf671-f03f-4d8d-b012-af79b633250e/.

17. Rose Kushner's Memorial, National Institutes of Health, January 30, 1990, Schlesinger Library, Harvard University.

18. Charles E. Rosenberg, *Explaining Epidemics and Other Studies in the History of Medicine* (New York: Cambridge University Press, 1992), 305.

19. "Actor Rock Hudson Has AIDS, Friend Says," *Cincinnati Post*, July 25, 1985, 12, https://www.newspapers.com/article/the-cincinnati-post-rocks-aidsreagan-r /153207955/.

20. "A Timeline of HIV and AIDS," U.S. Department of Health and Human Services, https://www.hiv.gov/hiv-basics/overview/history/hiv-and-aids-timeline/, accessed November 20, 2024; "Uncertainty Dominates Therapy for Breast Cancer," *Detroit Free Press*, September 5, 1981, 17, https://www.newspapers.com/article /detroit-free-press-1981-stats/154766915/.

21. "A Warning to Gay Men with AIDS," advertisement, *New York Native*, November 22, 1982, 16.

22. "A Timeline of HIV and AIDS."

23. Amy Sue Bix, "Diseases Chasing Money and Power: Breast Cancer and AIDS Activism Challenging Authority," *Journal of Public Policy* 9, special issue 1 (2011), https://www.cambridge.org/core/journals/journal-of-policy-history/article/abs /diseases-chasing-money-and-power-breast-cancer-and-aids-activism-challenging -authority/6D105E52016D95FA28B2D42F9FB56A35.

24. "Rock Hudson," Wikipedia, https://en.wikipedia.org/wiki/Rock_Hudson #Personal_life, accessed November 20, 2024.

25. Robert Shepard, "House Approves Millions for AIDS Research," UPI, October 3, 1985, https://www.upi.com/Archives/1985/10/03/House-approves-millions-for -AIDS-research/5541497160000/.

26. "Rock Hudson," Wikipedia.
27. Ibid.
28. "A Timeline of HIV and AIDS"; *The Phil Donahue Show,* March 18, 1985; "Breast Self Examination," *Lassen County Times,* November 26, 1985, https://www.newspapers .com/article/lassen-county-times-1985-bc-diagnoses/160301416/.
29. "A Timeline of HIV and AIDS."
30. Maia Szalavitz, "How to Survive a Plague: Q&A with ACT-UP's Peter Staley on Effective Activism," *Time,* September 27, 2012.
31. Samantha Vicenty, "How Princess Diana Changed the Way We Think About AIDS," *Oprah Daily,* November 27, 2020, https://www.oprahdaily.com /entertainment/tv-movies/a34550472/princess-diana-aids-charity-work/.
32. Pranay Gupte, "For Evelyn Lauder, the Past Is Certainly No Prologue," *New York Sun,* October 3, 2005, https://www.nysun.com/article/business-for-evelyn-lauder -the-past-is-certainly-no.
33. Susan Hirschhorn, phone interview with the author, October 23, 2023.
34. "2010 CSHL Double Helix Medals Dinner—Presented to Evelyn Lauder," YouTube, posted by Cold Spring Harbor Laboratory, July 23, 2013, https:// www.youtube.com/watch?v=yjaSWojUZ4o.
35. Ibid.
36. Ibid.
37. "Researchers Find Link Between Genetics and Breast Cancer," *Quad-City Times,* December 21, 1990, 3, https://www.newspapers.com/article/quad-city-times -king-identifies-chromoso/155045791/.
38. Ellen Elliott, "Women in Science: Mary-Claire King," Jackson Laboratory, February 27, 2017, https://www.jax.org/news-and-insights/jax-blog/2017/february /mary-claire-king#.
39. "Researchers Find Link Between Genetics and Breast Cancer."
40. Ibid.
41. Elliott, "Women in Science."
42. "Genetics Factor in How Long AIDS Patients Live," *Alabama Journal,* July 31, 1991, 5, https://www.newspapers.com/article/alabama-journal-mary-claire-king-and -aid/155094734/.
43. "*Self* (magazine)," Wikipedia, https://en.wikipedia.org/wiki/Self_ (magazine)#Editors-in-chief, accessed November 20, 2024.
44. "National Survey on Breast Cancer: A Measure of Progress in Public Understanding," National Institutes of Health, November 1980, 6, NIH Office of History.
45. Denise Flam, "Fashion's New Target,"*Newsday,* September 22, 1994, 121, https:// www.newspapers.com/article/newsday-nassau-edition-getting-press-f /157369532/.
46. Erica Geske, "How October and Pink Became Associated with Breast Cancer Awareness Month," Sullair, September 27, 2021, https://america.sullair.com/en /blog/how-october-pink-became-associated-breast-cancer-awareness-month.
47. Statement of Susan Ford Vance, chair of National Breast Cancer Awareness Program, Joint Hearing Before the Senate Subcommittee on Health and Long-Term Care and the Task Force on Social Security, and Women of the Select Committee on Aging, House of Representatives, 99th Congress, 1st Session, October 23, 1985, https://babel.hathitrust.org/cgi/pt?id=mdp .39015031727285&seq=25&q1=Vance.

Chapter 11

1. Sarah Handel and Michael Levitt, "Remembering Susan Love, Surgeon and Advocate for Breast Cancer Patients," *All Things Considered*, NPR, July 4, 2023, https://www.npr.org/2023/07/04/1185955988/remembering-susan-love-surgeon -and-advocate-for-breast-cancer-patients.
2. Susan Love in "Not Done: Women Remaking America," PBS, February 26, 2013, https://www.pbs.org/video/makers-women-who-make-america-dr-susan-love/.
3. Fran Visco, "Susan Love, a Transformative Leader in Breast Cancer Movement, Dies at 75," *Cancer Letter* 49, no. 27 (2023).
4. Nan Robertson, "A Woman's Crusade Against 'One-Step' Breast Surgery," *New York Times*, October 22, 1979, 6.
5. Susan M. Love, *Dr. Susan Love's Breast Book* (Cambridge, MA: Da Capo Press, 1990).
6. "Susan Love on Breast Cancer Activism in the 1990s," *Cancer History Project*, October 21, 2021, https://cancerhistoryproject.com/article/susan-love-on-breast-cancer -activism-in-the-1990s/.
7. James S. Olson, *Bathsheba's Breast: Women, Cancer and History* (Baltimore: Johns Hopkins University Press, 2004), 62.
8. Don Aucoin, "Approach to Breast Cancer Is Faulted," *Boston Globe*, May 13, 1991, 15, https://www.newspapers.com/article/the-boston-globe-bcc-organizes /155100474/.
9. Ibid.
10. Visco, "Susan Love."
11. Frances Chastain, "Why Research Is Poorly Funded," *The Republican*, May 2, 1991, 30, https://www.newspapers.com/article/the-republican-politics-of-bc-2/155096132/.
12. Olson, *Bathsheba's Breast*, 203.
13. "Pat Schroeder," Wikipedia, https://en.wikipedia.org/wiki/Pat_Schroeder, accessed November 20, 2024.
14. Ibid.
15. "National Women's History Month Spotlight: Former Congresswoman, Patricia Schroeder," *Joan's Blog*, https://www.joanlunden.com/category/33-joan-s-blog/item /145-national-women-s-history-month-spotlight-former-congresswoman-patricia -schroeder.
16. Michelle Green, "Pat Schroeder's Ambition to Be First Lady in the Oval Office Nears the Moment of Truth," *People*, September 7, 1987, https://people.com /archive/pat-schroeders-ambition-to-be-first-lady-in-the-oval-office-nears-the -moment-of-truth-vol-28-no-10/.
17. Bailey Vogt, "Pat Schroeder, Anita Hill's Former Adviser, Rebukes Joe Biden: 'He Wasn't Going to Let Her Testify,'" *Washington Times*, April 26, 2019, https://www .washingtontimes.com/news/2019/apr/26/pat-schroeder-anita-hills-former-adviser -rebukes-j/.
18. Statement of Anita Hill, professor, before the Committee on the Judiciary of the United States Senate, October 11, 1991, "Nomination of Judge Clarence Thomas to be Associate Justice of the Supreme Court of the United States," 102nd Congress, 1st Session.
19. "United States—Population: Population United States 1991," CountryEconomy .com, https://countryeconomy.com/demography/population/usa?year=1991.
20. Evelyn Lauder, ed., "*Self* Breast Cancer Report," *Self*, October 1991, 135.
21. Ibid., 136.

22. Ibid., 145.
23. Mary Ann Roser, "Letters to Congress Show Plight of Women with Breast Cancer," *Charlotte Observer,* October 9, 1991, 92, https://www.newspapers.com /article/the-charlotte-observer-write-thing-2-sc/48015954/.
24. Susan Ferraro, "The Anguished Politics of Breast Cancer," *New York Times Magazine,* August 15, 1993, 25.
25. "History of Women in the U.S. Congress," Center for American Women and Politics, Rutgers University, https://cawp.rutgers.edu/facts/levels-office/congress /history-women-us-congress, accessed November 20, 2024.
26. Ibid.
27. Judith L. Pearson, *From Shadows to Life: A Biography of the Cancer Survivorship Movement* (New York: Lincoln Square Books, 2021), 142.
28. Olsen, *Bathsheba's Breast,* 203.
29. "Letter Writers Seek Funds for Breast Cancer Research," *The Times* (Shreveport, LA), October 9, 1991, 37.
30. Katelyn Newman, "The Health Care Legacy of George H. W. Bush," *U.S. News and World Report,* December 5, 2018, https://www.usnews.com/news/national-news /articles/2018-12-05/george-hw-bushs-health-care-legacy.
31. "Coalition Demands Breast Cancer Funds," *Herald and Review,* July 28, 1991, 3.
32. Statement of Fran Visco, Joint Hearing Before the Select Committee on Aging and the Subcommittee on Health and Long-Term Care, 102nd Congress, 2nd Session, October 1, 1992, https://babel.hathitrust.org/cgi/pt?id=pst.000021236327&seq =108&q1=Visco&view=1up.
33. Roser, "Letters to Congress."
34. "Breast Cancer: Winning the Battles, Losing the War," second session of the 102nd Congress, statement of Fran Visco, joint hearing before the Select Committee on Aging and the Subcommittee on Health and Long-Term Care, https://babel .hathitrust.org/cgi/pt?id=pst.000021236327&seq=41&q1=minutes&view=1up.
35. "Voting: A Call to Arms," *Ventura County Star,* January 1, 1992, 40, https://www .newspapers.com/article/ventura-county-star-jan-1-voting-articl/156419680/.
36. Susan Hirschhorn, Zoom interview with the author, October 23, 2023.
37. "Narrowing the Field of Cosmetic Essentials," *Vancouver Sun,* April 2, 1992, 37, https://www.newspapers.com/article/the-vancouver-sun-desert-island-necessit /156370213/.
38. Robin Baker Leacock, *Mortimer's: A Moment in Time* (New York: G Editions, 2022).
39. "Princess Diana Talking to Liza Minnelli at the Sammy Davis Jr. Tribute Gala 1992," posted on the Liza with a Z Facebook page, March 1, 2019, https://www .facebook.com/watch/?v=2258556367748265.
40. Rob Scully, "Stars Salute Mr. Wonderful," *Reading Evening Post,* June 24, 1992, 7, https://www.newspapers.com/article/reading-evening-post-sammy-tribute -earni/158973737/.
41. "In Memoriam: Charlotte Haley, Creator of the First (Peach) Breast Cancer Ribbon," Breast Cancer Action, https://www.bcaction.org/in-memoriam -charlotte-haley-creator-of-the-first-peach-breast-cancer-ribbon/, accessed November 20, 2024.
42. Kathleen Hendrix, "Peach Corps," *Los Angeles Times,* August 20, 1992, https://www .latimes.com/archives/la-xpm-1992-08-20-vw-6473-story.html.
43. "In Memoriam: Charlotte Haley."
44. Alexandra Penney, phone interview with the author, September 18, 2024.

45. Ibid.
46. Ken Phillips, "The Color Pink—History, Meaning, and Facts," Hunter Lab, February 9, 2024, https://www.hunterlab.com/blog/the-color-pink/.
47. Eddie Coyle, "A Race with Many Winners," *New York Daily News*, October 14, 1991, 140.
48. U.S. Congress, "Joint Resolution to Designate October 1992, as 'National Breast Cancer Awareness Month,'" S.J. Res. 303, 102nd Congress, September 24, 1992.
49. Susan Hertog, "The War Against Breast Cancer: The Physician and the Lady," *Philanthropy Roundtable*, Fall 2016, https://www.philanthropyroundtable.org/magazine/the-war-against-breast-cancer/.
50. Eileen Nechas, *Unequal Treatment: What You Don't Know About How Women Are Mistreated by the Medical Community* (New York: Simon & Schuster, 1994), 86.
51. Ibid.
52. "Breast Cancer Coalition to Congress: 'Find a Way to Fund The War,' Bypass Level Is Not Enough," *Cancer Letter*, August 7, 1992, https://cancerhistoryproject.com/tcl-archive/19920807-1/.
53. "The Army Breast Cancer Research Program," introduction to *A Review of the Department of Defense's Program for Breast Cancer Research* (Washington, DC: National Academies Press, 1997), https://www.ncbi.nlm.nih.gov/books/NBK233671/.
54. "Vote Summary, Question: On the Amendment (Harkin Amdt No. 3142)," September 22, 1992, Roll Call Vote 102nd Congress, 2nd Session, https://www.senate.gov/legislative/LIS/roll_call_votes/vote1022/vote_102_2_00228.htm.
55. Olson, *Bathsheba's Breast*, 203.
56. Bonnie Erbe and Betsy Hart, "Was It the 'Year of the Woman?'" *Kenosha News*, November 7, 1992, 6, https://www.newspapers.com/article/kenosha-news-year-of-the-woman/156997364/.

Chapter 12

1. "Pretty as a Picture," *The Oregonian*, September 10, 1992, 28, https://www.newspapers.com/article/the-oregonian-evelyns-photos/156371267/.
2. Suzi Martin-Cusimano, "Cosmetics Queen Fights for Breast Cancer Cause," *Toronto Star*, October 15, 1992, 7, https://www.newspapers.com/article/the-toronto-star-info-on-ehl-center-and/156418937/.
3. Colette Bouchez, "Kettering Breast-Cancer Center Is State-of-the-Art," *New York Daily News*, September 30, 1992, 10, https://www.newspapers.com/article/daily-news-breast-center-opening-2/153804541/.
4. Ibid.
5. Susan Hertog, "The War Against Breast Cancer: The Physician and the Lady," *Philanthropy Roundtable*, Fall 2016, https://www.philanthropyroundtable.org/magazine/the-war-against-breast-cancer/.
6. Bouchez, "Kettering."
7. Sandra Morgan, *Into Our Own Hands: The Women's Health Movement in the United States, 1969-1990* (New Brunswick, NJ: Rutgers University Press, 2002), 126.
8. "Research Excludes Women, Study Says," *El Paso Times*, June 19, 1990, 5, https://www.newspapers.com/article/el-paso-times-gao-studywomen-in-researc/157135941/.

9. Eileen Nechas, *Unequal Treatment: What You Don't Know About How Women Are Mistreated by the Medical Community* (New York: Simon & Schuster, 1994), 22.

10. Ibid.

11. Ibid., 25.

12. Ibid., 26.

13. Hertog, "The War Against Breast Cancer."

14. Ibid.

15. Ibid.

16. Ibid.

17. Leonard Lauder, *The Company I Keep: My Life in Beauty* (New York: Harper Business, 2020), 336.

18. Mary Martin Niepold, "Action Defeats Dread," *Gloucester County Times,* October 24, 1993, 25, https://www.newspapers.com/article/gloucester-county-times-bcrf-2 /156367060/.

19. Breast Cancer Research Foundation press release, 1993, National Museum of American History, Smithsonian Institution.

20. Ibid.

21. Jana Petersen, "Ribbons Symbolize Breast Cancer Awareness," *St. Cloud Times,* October 13, 1993, 7, https://www.newspapers.com/article/st-cloud-times-bcrf -pink-ribbon-info/156366878/.

22. Denise Flaim, "Selling Social Consciousness," *Newsday,* October 28, 1993, 103, https://www.newspapers.com/article/newsday-nassau-edition-social-consciou /156367481/.

23. Ibid.

24. Petersen, "Ribbons"; "Mastectomy Photo Spurs Anger, Praise," *Daily Times* (Mamaroneck, NY), August 17, 1993, 3, https://www.newspapers.com/article /the-daily-times-bc-stats/154763882/.

25. Rose Kushner Oral History, Anne Kasper, interviewer, Kensington, MD, 1983, located at the Schlesinger Library, Harvard University.

26. Charter of the National Coalition for Cancer Survivorship, October 25, 1986, located at the NCCS archives in Silver Spring, MD.

27. Evelyn H. Lauder, *The Seasons Observed* (New York: Harry N. Abrams, 1994).

28. Baze Mpinja, "A Brief History of Estée Lauder Models," Yahoo Beauty, December 26, 2014, https://www.yahoo.com/lifestyle/a-brief-history-of-estee-lauder-models -104878623693.html.

29. "Black Versace Dress of Elizabeth Hurley," Wikipedia, https://en.wikipedia.org /wiki/Black_Versace_dress_of_Elizabeth_Hurley, accessed November 20, 2024.

30. "Actress to Shine as Estee Lauder Gal," *Fort Pierce Tribune,* March 9, 1995, 2, https:// www.newspapers.com/article/fort-pierce-tribune-hurley-selection /157497760/.

31. "Estée Lauder Lauds Elizabeth Hurley," *Fashion Week Daily,* April 11, 2008, https:// web.archive.org/web/20091021163932/http://www.fashionweekdaily .com/parties/fullstory.sps?inewsid=548687.

32. "Estee Lauder Companies and Elizabeth Hurley Talk About the Evolution of the Breast Cancer Campaign," YouTube, posted by New York Stock Exchange, October 14, 2023, https://www.youtube.com/watch?v=jEjqplUSRyk.

33. "*Charles: The Private Man, the Public Role,*" Wikipedia, https://en.wikipedia.org/wiki /Charles:_The_Private_Man,_the_Public_Role, accessed November 20, 2024.

34. Stephanie Petit, "The Real Story of Princess Diana's Revenge Dress," *People*, April 16, 2024, https://people.com/royals/princess-diana-revenge-dress-true-story/.

35. "Princess Diana Dress Auction 1997," posted on the Lady Diana Spencer Facebook page, July 24, 2021, https://www.facebook.com/watch/?v=2882439545352494.

36. Ibid.

37. Barbara McLaughlin, phone interview with the author, September 5, 2024.

38. "Catalogue, TV Bring Princess to Your Home," *Citizen Register*, June 25, 1997, 26, https://www.newspapers.com/article/citizen-register-auction-charities/154573542/.

39. "Princess Diana's Epic 1997 Dress Auction," *Eternal Goddess*, August 31, 2022.

40. "Princess Diana Dress Auction 1997."

41. "Diana Diaries: The 1997 Charity Dress Auction of 79 Dresses Worn by Princess Diana | People TV," YouTube, posted by People, September 16, 2020, https://www.youtube.com/watch?v=eZHfOmyMTnI.

42. James Sherwood, "Evelyn Lauder: Beauty Queen," *The Independent*, November 16, 2003, https://www.the-independent.com/news/people/profiles/evelyn-lauder-beauty-queen-78850.html.

43. Kyle Roderick, "Research Continues to Reduce Threat of Breast Cancer," *Rocky Mount Telegram*, October 19, 1998, 9, https://www.newspapers.com/article/rocky-mount-telegram-40-countries/157570678/.

44. "Breast Cancer: Are We on the Brink of Cure?," *Turlock Journal*, October 12, 1998, 7, https://www.newspapers.com/article/turlock-journal-1998-stats/157570297/.

45. Enid Nemy, "From Pink Lipstick to Pink Ribbons," *New York Times*, February 2, 1995, C1.

46. James S. Olson, *Bathsheba's Breast: Women, Cancer and History* (Baltimore: Johns Hopkins University Press, 2004), 7; "2000 Census: US Municipalities over 50,000: Ranked by 2000 Population," Demographia, https://demographia.com/db-uscity98.htm, accessed November 20, 2024.

47. Oliver Sacks, *A Leg to Stand On* (New York: Simon & Schuster, 1998), 7.

Epilogue

1. "About BCRF," Breast Cancer Research Foundation, https://www.bcrf.org/about, accessed November 20, 2024.

2. Julie Naughton and Pete Born, "Remembering Evelyn Lauder," *Women's Wear Daily*, November 12, 2011, https://wwd.com/business-news/human-resources/evelyn-lauder-dies-at-age-75-5365922/.

3. "Breast Cancer Facts and Stats," National Breast Cancer Foundation, last updated August 1, 2024, https://www.nationalbreastcancer.org/breast-cancer-facts/.

Index